# WOMAN'S OWN
## Book of
# Health & Beauty

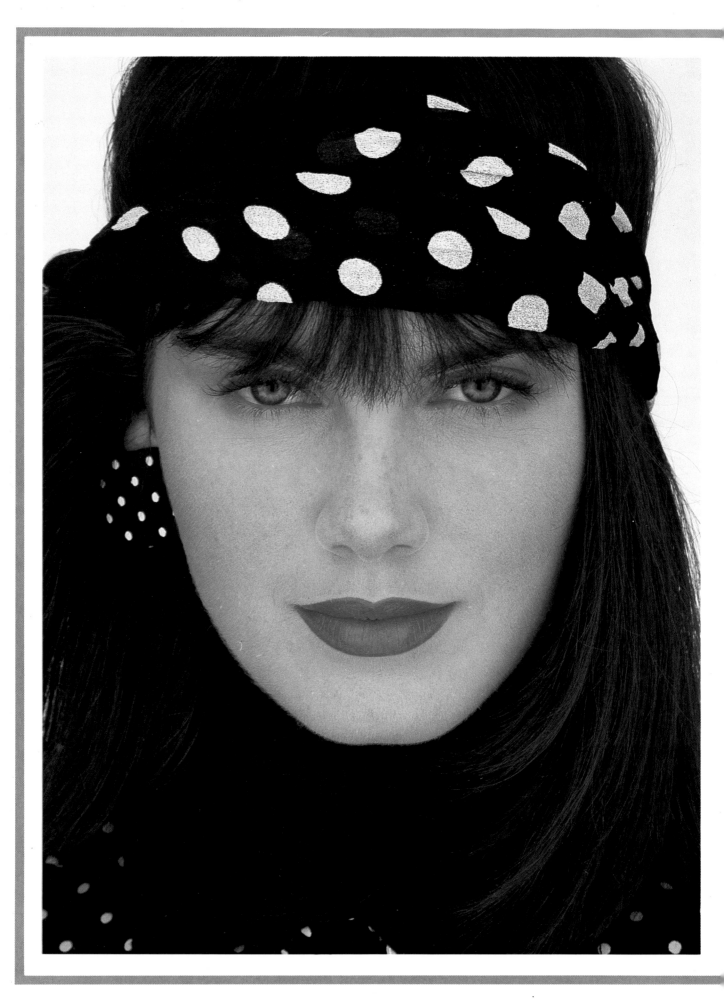

# WOMAN'S OWN
## Book of
# Health & Beauty

### Willa Beattie Wilson

**GUILD PUBLISHING**
LONDON

**Cover photography by Rob Lee**

Some of the material appearing in this book
was originally featured in *Woman's Own* magazine.

This edition published in 1986 by
Book Club Associates
by arrangement with The Hamlyn Publishing Group Limited
Bridge House, London Road, Twickenham, Middlesex, England.

Phototypeset in England by Photocomp Limited
in 10 on 12pt Palatino.

Printed in Spain

# Contents

# Introduction

*Woman's Own has been a great magazine for more than 50 years and its beauty pages have always been leaders in their field – fun, informative and factual. We're particularly proud of our reader relationship – our down-to-earth diets, our Fun Run and our fabulous reader make-overs. In this first-ever* Woman's Own *Beauty Book you'll find all you need to know about make-up, skin care, health and hair, plus a once-and-for-all diet and fascinating information from some of the world's most attractive women on the beauty routines that work for them. I know you'll enjoy it.*

*Bridget Rowe*

BRIDGET ROWE
Editor, *Woman's Own*

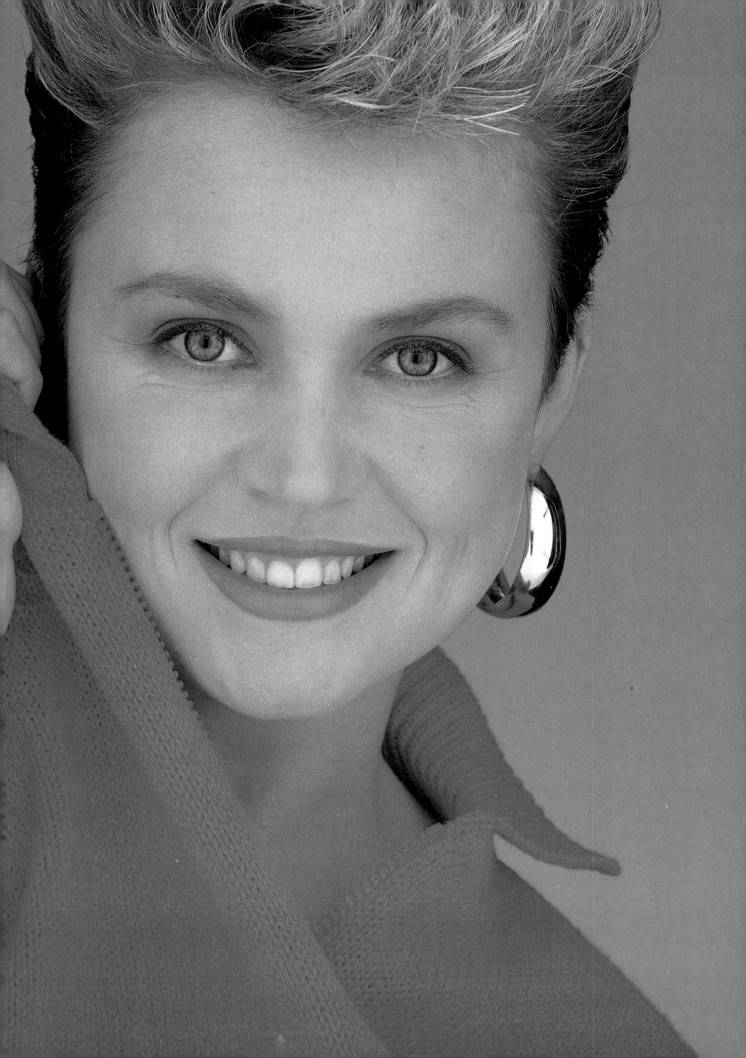

# Skin Care

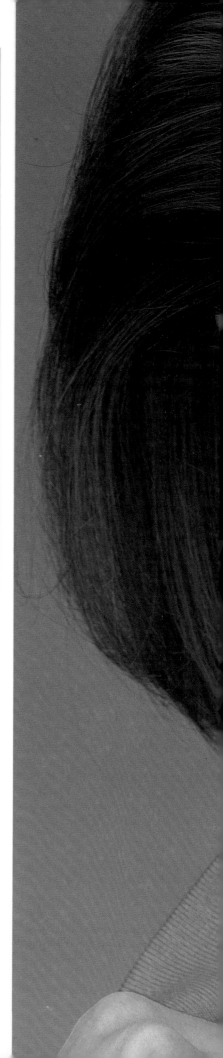

*Perfect skin should be firm, yet elastic and full of glowing vitality. With a little care and attention, we can all aspire to this pinnacle of perfection.*

*Whatever your skin type, it will give warning signals when it's being badly treated. Lines may develop slowly, but sudden illness or too much of the good life can leave skin looking dull and strained. An understanding of your skin plus a regular, but never obsessive, care routine can contain many problems and modern treatments can improve and prolong skin's youthful complexion. To keep skin looking good, a daily cleansing and moisturizing routine is essential.*

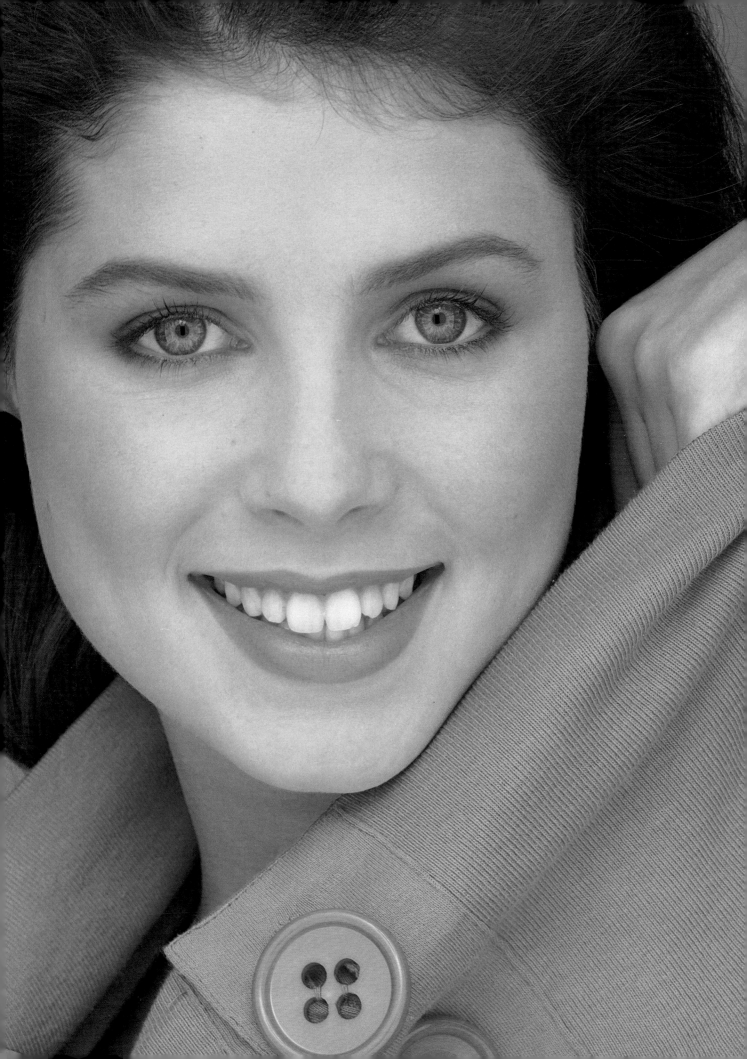

# Skin – the glowing asset

First, we must understand how skin operates and how it is likely to react not only to age, diet and stress, but to environmental conditions, such as centrally heated offices, wind and sun.

Skin is made up of protective layers of cells supported by nerves, glands and blood vessels. In a continual process, cells work their way to the surface where they are shed and replaced. This top layer is protected and smoothed naturally by oils and water excreted from the sebaceous sweat glands.

On reaching the skin's surface, the water evaporates and leaves a fine film of protective oil, a balancing act which is regulated by our hormones. Skin, which has a slightly acidic natural pH balance of 6·5, dries out when the glands don't produce enough oily lubrication to prevent excessive water evaporation. Conversely, when the oil glands are over-stimulated, they produce too much oil which gathers under the skin's surface and clogs pore openings. The trapped oil irritates the surrounding skin and inflammation results.

Top dermatologists agree that the condition of your skin is largely a matter of hormones and inheritance, but internal and external factors over which we do have some control can also affect skin.

Internal factors affecting skin include hormones, diet, stress, bad circulation, lack of exercise, smoking, alcohol and drugs. External factors like hot and cold weather, strong winds and air conditioning can also upset the skin's balance, depriving it of its essential moisture. The drier the air, the more the skin loses its own natural water supply. Particularly in winter when the central heating is on, you only have to look at your droopy plants or dried-out woodwork to realize that the heating is burning up valuable moisture. You may also notice that you receive static electricity shocks from carpeting and door knobs. These are signals that there is a relative drop in humidity, causing skin cells to shrink, giving a rough-to-touch feel. All skins need moisture, even oily skin, so it's well worth investing in a heavier moisturizer to top up, and inexpensive humidifiers to hang on radiators throughout winter. They will help the moisture balance, but do remember to fill them regularly with fresh water and change the filters when they look dirty.

# What's your skin type?

**Normal** skin is soft and supple to touch. This is due to a perfect balance of the natural lubricating water and oil mixture.

Normal skin still needs a regular daily routine of cleansing, toning and moisturizing and a monthly facial – cleaning out or simply pepping up with a face mask. It may 'break out' as a result of hormonal changes before or during menstruation or excessive sunbathing, so be prepared to give it some extra special care and treatment at these times.

Sensible eating, sleeping and relaxation all work indirectly to improve the skin's condition.

**Combination skin** is easy to identify. You may notice, a few hours after you've applied your make-up, that your nose, forehead and chin start to shine. You only have to do the tissue test: blot your face with a tissue and hold it up to the light, to find impregnated oily panels down the centre. Spots or blackheads are only likely to appear around this oily panel. The answer is to double up on some of your cleansing toning and moisturizing products. Use a lighter moisturizer around the greasy panel but, more important, opt for an oatmeal scrub or mask to clean out the centre clogged pores, being careful to avoid cheek areas which don't need such rigorous and abrasive cleansing.

**Oily skin,** although irritating when it tends to shine minutes after you've finished applying your make-up, is less susceptible to wrinkles, lines and old age because it is *naturally* well lubricated with oils. Unfortunately, it makes for a sallow complexion, tends to have over-active oil glands which produce visible coarse open pores, and is susceptible to blackheads and spots. A *strict* cleansing régime is the way to keep oily skin looking fresh, bright and spot-free. Lightweight facial masks (see pages 26 to 27) can be used once a week, although some French dermatologists say that a daily mask or liquid facial scrub can do no harm. You could try the dermatological facial bars, which are *not* soap detergents, to give your face a real feeling of freshness.

**Dry skin** is a typical Anglo-Saxon phenomenon. Dry skin is generally fair, fine, small-pored, and slightly sensitive. It flakes and peels easily, and feels taut and tight after washing with normal soap and water. It's the first to show the early signs of fine lines around eyes and mouth and is particularly vulnerable to the elements – central heating and sun. The sebaceous oil glands tend to be underactive – not supplying enough lubrication.

All skin types dry naturally as we get older due to a slowing down of the hormones and metabolism but if you are born with a dry skin, then you are never *too* young to learn the art of prevention and protection. Opt for a gentle cleansing and heavier moisturizing routine but don't forget that your skin, particularly if you live in a city, still needs the once-a-month clean-out.

Fortunately, there are now many products on the market to cope with

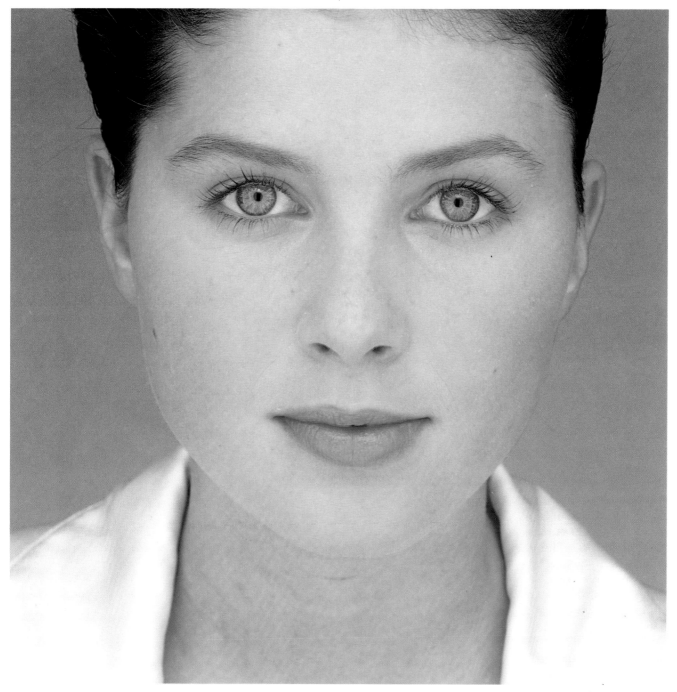

dry skins. These range from enriched cleansing milks to regenerated ampules or oils (either the old aromatheraphy essential oils or the newer collagen serums which actually filter through the hair follicles, through the top skin layer and 'plump up' the cells helping to regenerate the tissues and giving the skin a smoother appearance). There are also professional treatments by a method called 'Iontophoresis' which introduces oil into the skin via a galvanic current. It's painless and temporarily effective for dry skin.

**Sensitive skin,** also dry, is the most delicate. It looks translucent, is prone to freckles, blotches, broken veins, dermatitis, and is allergic to many ingredients in cosmetic products. The worst enemy for dry, sensitive skin is dehydration: it makes skin feel tight, look dull and lifeless, and vulnerable to dry facial

*With the correct skin care, everyone can have healthy, glowing skin.*

lines. Skin irritations flare up quickly so it is easy to detect which product is the culprit. There are many hypo-allergenic products on the market, which are usually fragrance-free, and are formulated to eliminate many of the known irritants like lanolin, colouring agents, alcohol and preservatives.

Fragrance is the major offender; remember that your neck is just as sensitive as your face and avoid dousing yourself in perfume. There's also no guarantee, just because a product promises to be hypo-allergenic, that your skin still won't react violently, so buy smaller bottles in the range and test on small skin patches, such as inside elbow, until you find the skin-care range that your skin is happiest with. If your skin feels itchy or comes up in a red patch, stop using the product immediately, give your skin a rest, and go back to trial and error. Remember that household soap and detergents can trigger off eczema, severe cases of which should be medically treated.

## Skin-care routine: day care

Clear skin that gleams with healthy colour and has an even texture can only result from daily attention. The simple but vital key to good skin care is cleanliness – removing grime, excess oils, perspiration, make-up – *twice* daily. Cleaning up is not stripping the skin but gently removing the surface debris. And there's nothing wrong with soap and water if you don't feel clean without.

### Soaps and cleansers
Even sensitive skins can take soap of the fragrance-free type. The days of the harsh alkaline soaps which strip the skin of its natural oils are over. Today's market offers non-alkaline soaps, complexion bars or soapless soaps which don't form a scum even in hard water. But soaps will only clean; they can't actually moisturize the skin since they are rinsed off the skin's surface. Another problem is that most soaps will *not* remove stubborn make-up so they are best used in the morning.

Now we are seeing soaps which are, paradoxically, soap-free! Vichy's Aqua-Tendre dermatological cleansing bar, guaranteed soap-free, is ideal for delicate, sensitive skins. It contains 'surface active' cleansing agents as opposed to soaps' alkaline detergent. The Body Shop's raspberry scented tablet Milk Protein Cleansing Bar is based on syndet – a synthetic substitute for soap. Roc's Compact Facial Cleanser is also a new concept – it's neither a soap nor a cleansing bar but a solidified hypoallergenic and perfume-free cleansing milk that you use with water. All these products are neutral pH balanced.

'Soapy' cleansers also come in the form of liquid soaps and cleansing milks which are light, fluffy, water-based and easily rinsed off.

Heavier-duty cleansers tend to be greasier and should be removed with damp pads of cotton wool (much kinder to the skin than tissues). Make sure you get into the crevices around nose and eyes.

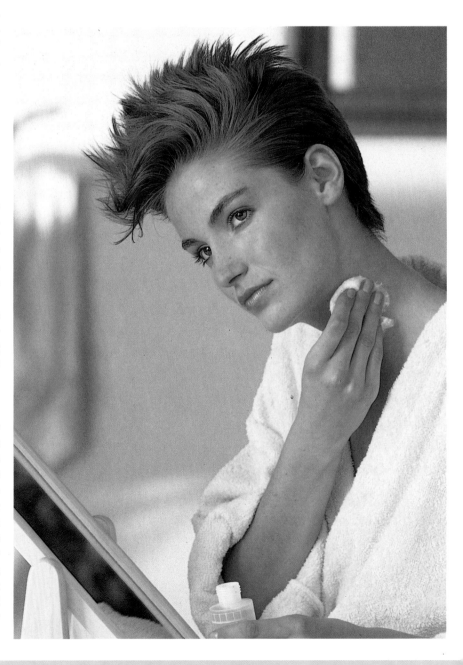

## Toners, fresheners or astringents

These remove the last traces of these cleansing agents and will go further if you apply them with slightly damp cotton pads. Their astringent properties boost the skin's circulation, tighten the pores and provide a pleasant 'morning fresh' feeling.

To see if your skin is thoroughly cleansed, one of the simplest spot checks is to wipe your face with a pad of cotton wool dampened with water and witch-hazel, using the edges of the pad to wipe in the creases at the sides of nose and centre of chin. Check the pad for any signs of dirt.

## Moisturizers

Morning moisturizers should be suited to your skin type and be lighter than night creams. Remember, you don't want tight, taut skin nor do you want a greasy face to start the day. You want smooth, moisturized, clean skin – the perfect canvas for make-up. If your skin tends to be oily then opt for one of the specially formulated under-base moisturizers for a fine protective film. If you want to show off clear skin without any foundation then try some of the tinted moisturizers for a healthy glow.

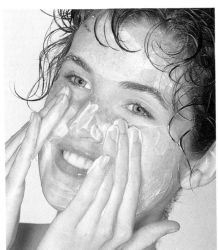

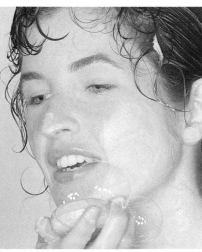

*Some women don't feel their skin's clean with a soap-and-water wash. Others feel their skin's too sensitive to take anything but the gentlest cleanser. However, today there are 'soapy' cleansers which are gentle on the skin and can be rinsed off.*

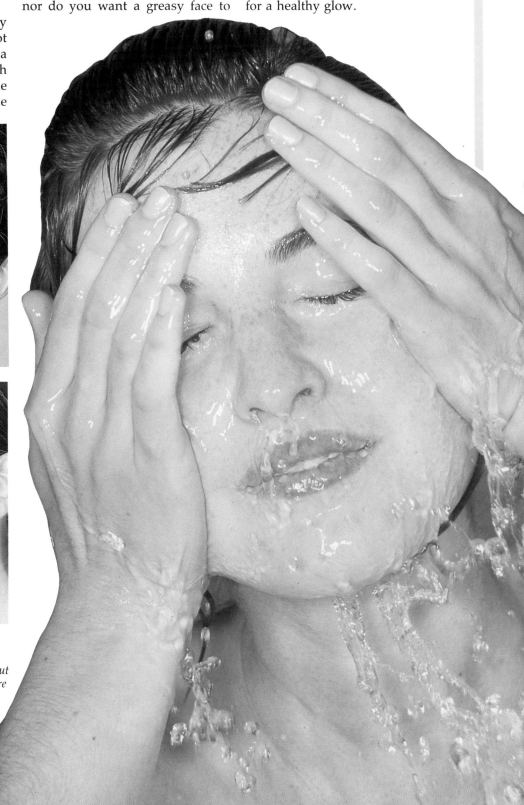

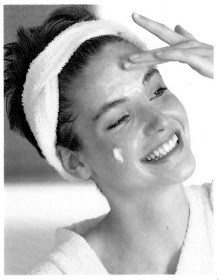

## Skin care routine: night care

A meticulous session at night to remove the last traces of make-up is essential and remember that your moisturizer is a must. Moisturizers come in various forms and textures and all attempt to replace water and oil when our natural supply needs a boost. It's never too late or too early to help skin along with creams, lotions and oils.

There are basically two things that we need from a skin cream. Firstly, we want to make our skin 'normal' – less dry or less greasy. And secondly, we want to stave off wrinkles for as long as possible.

Night care is vitally important. While we sleep we can give our skin a rest from make-up and outside environmental factors, and give it a boost with the right moisturizer.

**A good moisturizer should:**

● add water into the upper layers of the skin and keep it there for as long as possible.

● slow down moisture loss by putting a semi-occlusive barrier (a sort of raincoat) on top of the skin.

● protect skin from premature ageing by screening the sun's rays.

Moisturizers should also be pleasant to use. Thicker creams do slow down the skin's own natural water loss but some are so heavy they smear over your neckline or pillow.

The nicest ones to use are water-based (sometimes called oil-in-water), which are light enough to be absorbed quickly into your skin. Usually they're in lotion form and runny rather than solid. Until the 1950s, before this formula was discovered by Dr Nathan Black, an American dermatologist, all moisturizers had been greasy and unpleasant to use because they were oil-based. (Oils alone cannot moisturize skin; they can only lock in water.)

The search is now on for new ingredients or new formulations of old ones, to make a pleasant-to-use moisturizer that will last for several hours. Meanwhile, world-wide skin-care companies have launched intensive seven and 14-day night

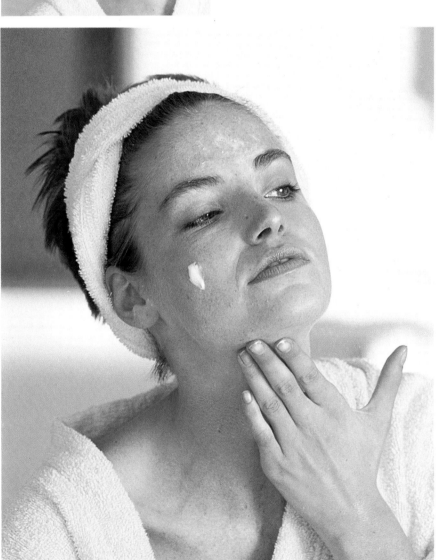

*Dry areas like cheeks need extra conditioning. Eye creams stop tiny lines, and don't forget that throats can give away your age as quickly as your eyes, so cleanse and moisturize these areas as you would your face.*

treatments for repairs to skin that has excessively dried out.

## Dry skin: new ingredients

One of the more exciting developments in skin creams is the discovery of a polymer called polyglyceryl methacrylate as a moisturizing agent.

A major supplier of raw materials for cosmetics believes that polymer genuinely acts as a moisture barrier – and is more effective than collagen, elastin, and plant extracts.

Another significant discovery is the moisturizing properties of glycerine. Glycerine is a humectant, which means that it hangs on to water and stops evaporation from the skin. It has long been used in nourishing creams, but made them heavy and sticky to use. Recent formulas have made glycerine much more refined and acceptable.

Several leading skin-care manufacturers are now using the above-mentioned ingredients in their moisturizers. But until ingredients are listed on beauty product packaging (as they are in the USA), we will not know which creams contain what. Most manufacturers keep their formulas secret, but we do know that Avon's Night Support (a fluid which claims to help the skin to repair itself overnight), contains polyglyceryl methacrylate. And Pond's Cream and Cocoa Butter Lotion contain glycerine.

## Greasy skin: the way ahead

Progress hasn't been as good for those with greasy skins as for those with dry ones. The search is still on for creams that don't add grease, and we're still a long way from finding any that can mop up existing greasiness. Scientists are also searching for products that will enable sebum (the oil), to be removed effectively from the sebaceous glands. It is probably best to opt for an oil-free moisturizer which fools the sebaceous glands into thinking they've been moisturized and then curbs their instinct to do overtime after you've washed your face. Don't forget that neck and eye areas should still be treated to a moisturizer after washing or cleansing your face.

## Stopping the clock

Can we look 40 at 50? And if so, how? One of the biggest breakthroughs is the incorporation of UV-B filters in daytime skin-care products which can stop the harmful rays at a level of 50 per cent. More and more moisturizers, and even foundations and bases, now contain these effective filters. (see tanning, page 138)

## Wrinkles

Certain products even claim they can undo ageing damage, such as the start of tiny facial lines and crows' feet, after it has begun. Estée Lauder's Prescriptives Line Preventor is a lightweight fluid which you apply under moisturizer twice a day.

It makes the appealing claim of preventing the visible aspects of ageing, at source, before they occur. The theory is that your skin ages when groups of molecules called free radicals cause cells not to reproduce properly. Prescriptives Line Preventor, it is claimed, stops these free radicals from doing their damage. It's hard to judge from testing because you don't know what your skin would have looked like if you hadn't used it! Still, it's an interesting concept, as yet unproven.

## False economy

Just because a moisturizer is expensive doesn't mean it is good, but cosmetic scientists do say that most cheap moisturizers consist simply of mineral oils, lanolin and wax, or mineral oils and petroleum jelly. They warn that petroleum jelly stops the skin from breathing and inflames sweat glands, and mineral oils don't stimulate the natural oils of the skin very well.

In general, plant oils do this better than mineral oils, they cost more. A good moisturizer containing effective protective oils, hydrating agents and a sunscreen will be in the middle price range.

If your funds are limited, economize on your cleanser since this just removes impurities and you can opt for a cold water splash to close pores rather than an expensive toner. Then you can put the money you've saved towards a better moisturizer.

---

### Skin-care summary

**Oily skin:** remove cosmetics in the evening with a cleansing lotion or skin oil. Apply toner or a heavier astringent. Use a lighter all-over moisturizer and invest in special products for neck and eye areas, especially if you are over 30.

**Dry and sensitive skin:** Use a light cleansing cream, freshener and moisturizer. Concentrate on delicate eye area with a cream specifically refined for the job and invest in a heavier duty throat cream. (Sensitive skins are happiest with fragrance-free, hypoallergenic products.)

**Combination skin:** Treat your face as oily down the centre T panel, and dry on cheeks, neck and around eyes.

**Normal skin:** Remove make-up with cream or lotion. Apply toner, then moisturizer where necessary (in the neck and eye areas usually).

All skins are individual. If a consultant suggests other treatments for you, follow her advice.

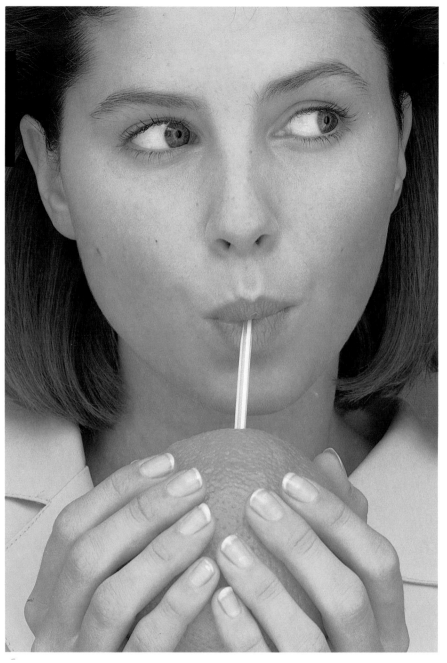

DAY 1 – choose from:

### Beetroot bonus

A glass of beetroot juice will cleanse the liver, the kidneys and improve the quality of your blood, building up the red corpuscles. To make two glasses, blend 8oz/225g scrubbed, or peeled, grated carrot with 4oz/100g beetroot, 2fl oz/3 table-spoon apple juice and $\frac{1}{2}$ to $\frac{3}{4}$ pint/300 to 450ml water.

### Cleansing carrots

If you've over-indulged in food and wine, carrot juice will alkalize an acid system and contains B-complex vitamins a well as A, C, E and K. To make one glass blend 4oz/100g scrubbed, grated carrot with $\frac{1}{8}$ pint/ 4 tablespoons apple juice and top up with water to taste. For a sav-oury version, blend carrot with 1 stick celery, 1 tablespoon natural yogurt, 1 teaspoon vinegar, black pepper and $\frac{1}{4}$ pint/150ml water.

### Sweet watercress

Watercress is a powerful diuretic and contains a large amount of sulphur as well as iodine. To make one glass, blend 1 bunch trimmed watercress with $\frac{1}{3}$ pint/200ml apple juice. Top up with water to taste.

## Two-day drinking spree for skin

What you eat and drink is reflected in your looks. Because skin needs nourishment internally as well as externally, try our two-day drinking spree to detoxify the system and give your skin the extra boost it needs after an indulgent holiday or the Christmas season.

Choose any one of the first four drinks on Day 1, sipping about $\frac{1}{3}$ pint every three to four hours. On Day 2 choose one of the next six drinks, according to your body and your taste buds, and drink the same quantity. Use fizzy or still mineral water to top up your glass to taste. Note: you will need a liquidizer or blender to make these drinks.

IMPORTANT: Remember, before embarking on any diet, be sure to check your general health with your doctor first. See our own diet plans on page 60 to 69.

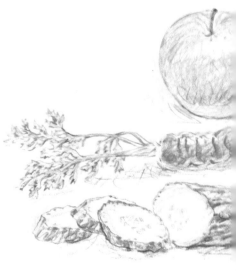

## Vegetable delight

For one glass, blend together 5 or 6 lettuce leaves, 2 sticks of trimmed celery, 1 tablespoon fresh parsley, 1 tomato, 1 tablespoon malt vinegar, pepper and $\frac{1}{4}$ pint/150 ml water or more to taste. Together, these ingredients will work to expel extra fluid in your body.

DAY 2 – choose from:

## Body booster

If you suffer from pre-menstrual tension then your body is high on sodium and low on phosphates. Two foods that will help to re-establish a natural balance of these substances are avocado and banana. For one glass, blend 1 banana with $\frac{1}{4}$ pint/150 ml skimmed milk, 1 table-spoon lemon juice and a pinch of nutmeg. Alternatively, blend half a peeled avocado with a squeeze of lemon juice, 1 in/2·5 cm chunk peeled cucumber, $\frac{1}{2}$ tablespoon fresh parsley, black pepper and $\frac{1}{4}$ pint/150 ml water.

## Coconut goodness

The coconut is highly nutritious with vitamins B and C, protein and natural oils. For one glass, blend milk from 1 coconut with $\frac{1}{4}$ pint/ 150 ml skimmed milk, $\frac{1}{4}$ coconut flesh, peeled and grated, and 1 teaspoon runny honey. Drink chilled.

## Fruity salad cocktail

Concoct your own fruit juice with your special favourites. For two glasses, blend 1 peeled banana, 1 cored apple and 1 peeled and pip-ped orange with 2 tablespoons natural yogurt and water to taste. Add other fruit if desired.

## Ice-cool melon

Melons are full of vitamins A and C and have superb natural sweetness. On the hottest days melon blended and diluted with mineral water makes the most refreshing, cooling drink. For one glass, blend 6 oz/ 175 g peeled melon, $\frac{1}{2}$ teaspoon ground ginger and 2 tablespoons fresh orange juice. Serve in a long glass with crushed ice.

## Mango magic

The mango is packed with vitamins A and C, potassium, calcium, phos-phorus and magnesium. When in the sun, Vitamin A will protect you against the effects of excessive de-hydration. For one glass, blend $\frac{1}{4}$ peeled mango with 2 tablespoons lemon juice, $\frac{1}{3}$ pint/200 ml apple juice and water to taste.

## Pineapple power

Apart from plenty of vitamin C, pineapple contains an enzyme which aids digestion. For one glass, blend $\frac{1}{2}$ lb/225 g peeled ripe fresh pineapple with $\frac{1}{4}$ pint/150 ml water and a dash of fresh orange juice.

# Spotting the problems

Perfect skin is rare. Very few of us can boast that we haven't broken out in the odd spot or two occasionally or seen the first signs of red veins or strange lumps and bumps. They may seem minor but when they appear on the face or neck, common skin blemishes can ruin your looks.

**Spots** are the most common skin complaint. Most dermatologists define spots as either a mild outcrop of spots or a severe case of spots (not acne), caused by the inheritance of a greasy, spot-prone skin and the circulating male hormones present in all our bodies.

Most cases of major spot eruption occur at puberty when the body is going through enormous physical and hormonal changes. When these go slightly out of balance, the male hormones cause the sebaceous glands to secrete excessive amounts of oil. These outbreaks usually show on the face, back and chest because there are more sebaceous glands in these areas than other parts of the body. Other instances of hormone imbalance that can trigger off spots occur during the early stages of pregnancy and the menopause.

We actually have more than 2,000 oil glands per square inch of skin. When the sebum (oil) builds up, causing a blockage, a chemical reaction with bacteria occurs in the upper part of the hair follicle. This in turn produces highly irritating fatty acids which battle below the skin's surface and build up into an angry red bump on the surface, usually inflamed.

Never pick your spots – you'll only spread infection. It's best to see your doctor who will, if necessary, arrange for you to see a dermatologist. Treatment usually consists of mildly abrasive cleansing to open the exit line for the trapped sebum. Sometimes antibiotics are prescribed. Acned skin can leave permanent scarring and a pitted surface so leave it to the experts.

If you just have the odd spot, keep it clean with an antiseptic cream and cleanse it well so that the new cells can move quickly upwards. A steam facial, which opens the pores, is one of the best ways to encourage spots to the surface. You can conceal spots with antiseptic camouflage tinted sticks which dry out the spot and still allow you to wear foundation or base. Never leave make-up on a spot-prone skin: cleanse . . . cleanse . . . cleanse.

**Blackheads** are more likely to occur if you have an oily or combination skin where excess oil is continually clogging up the surface. They are not dirt but simply clogged-up compact masses of sebum which attract bacteria. Remove them with a steam facial and gently extract by pressing, *never* by squeezing.

**Open pores** are likely to occur on greasy/combination skin. Pores are stretched because of the excess of oil flow but they can be kept under control by scrupulous cleansing and toning. Toning helps temporarily, whereas face packs and masks give more lasting help to refine enlarged pores.

**Whiteheads** are raised bumps under the skin's surface, often associated with an acidic skin and a weight problem. A professional beauty therapist can easily remove these but don't attempt to pick at them with a needle yourself – you could damage surrounding skin and scar your face.

**Broken veins** are usually found around cheekbones and are more common on fine, delicate and sensitive skins. They are not actually broken but dilated capillaries. They can be aggravated by extremes of temperature, harsh treatments, hot spicy foods, smoking and excess alcohol. A beauty therapist can remove them by cauterizing the capillary (spideruein) with a fine needle in a method similar to electrolysis. This is one of the commoner skin problems experienced by people with fair, Anglo-Saxon looks.

To prevent these blemishes from appearing, use gentle products on the skin, avoid extremes of heat and cold and *always* wear protective moisturizer with UV filters if you're sitting in the sun or playing a sport. And don't forget that even sitting under a hairdrier can aggravate the skin, so take along your moisturizer. If you only need to camouflage slightly, see page 17.

**Sebaceous cysts** are caused by a blockage in the sebaceous duct but can easily be removed medically by means of a small incision; the lump then usually pops out like a pea in a pod. Always see your doctor as soon as the lump appears.

**Moles** can be attractive but if they are large, raised and unsightly with hairs growing from them it doesn't necessarily mean that they are harmful. Never try to pick the hairs from a mole with tweezers: it can make the mole look even larger (you can cut the hair with scissors). Always have moles checked by a doctor first she may suggest a dermatological treatment such as planing off the skin's surface and having the hair expertly removed by electrolysis.

**Warts** are caused by a virus similar to the verucca. Often seen on the hands, they occasionally appear on the face and either disapper on their own or may be burned out with chemicals. But as all the rogue cells have to be destroyed without harming the surrounding area, before you decide to do it yourself, check with a doctor.

**Wrinkles** are caused by the ageing process that takes place in the dermis, just under the top layer of skin. They appear firstly under the eyes and around the upper lip. It is now possible to postpone the ageing process (see pages 156 to 159).

**Age spots or brown spots** are part of the ageing process (see page 157).

**Skin tags** often appear on the neck in later life. Harmless pieces of extra skin, sometimes resembling small warts, they can be removed by means of electrolysis.

## Do-it-yourself facials

### Exfoliation

It doesn't matter how much money you spend on your moisturizer, it won't be able to do its job unless your skin is receptive to treatment. Dermatologists have been lecturing us for years on the importance of exfoliation – sloughing off top dead skin cells. We renew our skin cells by the minute but it normally takes within 20 to 28 days to replace the superficial top layer totally. If these cells don't lift off, skin can look dull and grey. They also hinder the skin's ability to eliminate wastes and produce a regular flow of oil and water. If these can't surface, you can't expect your moisturizer to penetrate. You may have thought that grandmother's skin looked okay on good ol' soap and water and didn't need these complicated techniques, but in fact she was probably doing a perfect job of exfoliation by using rougher flannels than the ones we use today.

**The range of products** available today means we can enjoy our luxury lines in towels and flannels and whisk off dead skin with the latest forms of scrubs – creams and cleansers which have tiny granules in them to lift off dead skin cells gently. There are also soaps with natural oatmeal grains in them or you can buy beauty grains and mix them with water to form a paste for washing yourself.

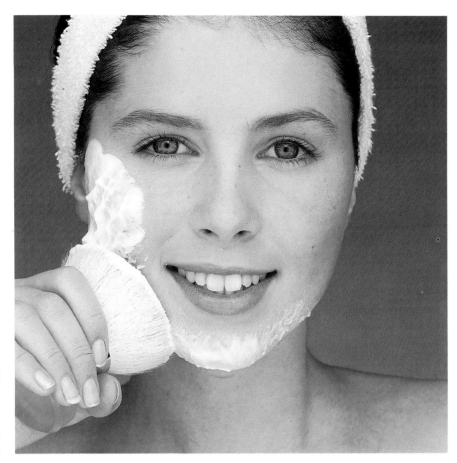

For extra sensitive skin it may be better to lather up using a pH balanced soap, and then removing the dead surface cells using a soft shaving brush with a circular motion. Creamy masks are also effective (see page 27). Dry skins tend to have flaky, patchy spots so opt for a rich, creamy scrub that washes off easily with warm water. Oily skins need a good basic clean-up but scrubbing often hinders, since this will only stimulate and overactivate the oil glands. Sensitive skins need allergy-tested, fragrance-free scrubs like those in the Clinique range.

**When and how often** you decide to give your skin the rub depends on your own particular skin type. Study your skin closely using a magnifying mirror under a light to see if you can spot any scaly patches or clogged up pores and blackheads. Scrubs do a wonderful job of cleaning out and preparing the skin for other treatments.

*If you have a sensitive skin exfoliate with a soapy lather and soft shaving brush.*

Dry and sensitive skins would benefit more from a nightly treatment since you want to let your skin breathe and if it's particularly sensitive you may find it will react to putting on make-up straight away. Don't have a facial on the day you're going out for an important date: you could end up with a red face!

Before scrubbing, it's best to give your face a steam bath. Fill a bowl with boiling water, add a drop or two of your favourite essential oil, bend over the bowl with a towel for several minutes. The steam opens up the pores and makes it easier to remove the trapped grime. Wipe over the face with cotton wool. Once you've cleaned out you should close the pores by splashing your face with cold water, or give yourself a moisturizing mask (see page 26).

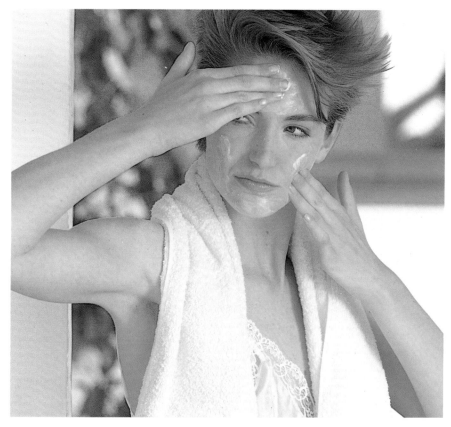

## Massage

Massage not only cleanses and conditions; it also raises the skin's temperature and improves blood circulation. Facial massage is good for all skin types, providing it is done gently and in the right direction.

Every professional facial at a salon after routine cleansing, exfoliation, blackhead and whitehead removal, masks and conditioning, finishes with a few minutes face and neck massage which is probably the most relaxing part.

**The most popular methods** of massage include Swedish massage and Shiatsu. The Swedish technique involves a more vigorous and stimulating method of kneading, stroking, rolling and squeezing than Shiatsu which works on the acupuncture points using fingers and thumb.

**Aromatherapy** is a revived art using natural plant oils. Essential oils are massaged onto the skin using a combination of acupressure, Shiatsu and Swedish massage. Aroma-

*Try to find time once a week to give your face a massage following the easy steps opposite page. This method is used in Elizabeth Arden salons.*

therapy is used to treat nervous disorders, fluid retention, sinus complaints and wrinkles. A favourite beauty treatment at many salons and health farms, it can be used either on the face or body but the oils and treatment are expensive.

**Home massage** There are many techniques used in facial massage but here are a few simple guidelines so you can give yourself a face-lifting massage at home.

A massage which exerts *slight* pressure is ideal for beginners: never tug or pull at skin: be gentle yet firm. If you want your skin to absorb oils and creams in a treatment, start with clean skin. If you love the freshness of herbs, use an essential oil for slicker lubrication. Tie or wrap hair away from neck and face.

**Neck and shoulders** Start at the neck and shoulder area where a lot of tension builds up. Using both hands place right hand on centre of chest and sweep upwards and outwards over to the left side of neck and shoulders. Repeat with left hand on right side of chest and alternate movements in a steady rhythmic motion.

Ease tension at back of neck, again with both hands. Cup hands into the contours of neck, one at the bottom of neck and the other at the base of skull. Pull each hand lightly up from base of neck to back of skull, alternating hands in this upward pull. Follow on by moving around the neck, first bringing one hand and then the other around the neck curve from back to front.

On front of neck, chest and up towards throat, use finger pads in upward and outward strokes to jaw line.

**Face** Moving to your face, start on chin line to relax jaw and trim chin. Put thumbs under centre of chin-line and stroke outwards towards end of jaw line. Work on centre of chin. Using fingertips and pads press and push chin gently upwards and outwards to ears. Try a methodical movement using both hands and gradually move upwards on each side from mouth corners in a sweep across to ear lobes.

Never massage the eyesocket area since this tends to be delicate and lacks strong muscle power. Start from centre of eyebrows and move across and around the eye area in one circular movement to bridge of nose. Never tug eye area underneath or above against this natural oval. Massage on the eye area is best left to the experts.

Relax and discourage frown lines on the forehead with two simple techniques. Start by working across from the centre above eyebrows to each side, sliding fingertips across to hairline above the ear. Gradually move up until the whole forehead has been crossed to temples. Next use fingers in a vertical direction, gently sliding upwards from eyebrows to hairline. Never pull frown lines down – always ease across or upwards.

A tension releaser at the temples can easily be manipulated with pads of fingers. Slowly massage temples in a circular movement, lightly to begin with and then gradually exerting slight pressure.

Put on your favourite music, close your eyes and relax for 10 minutes.

# Step-by-step massage

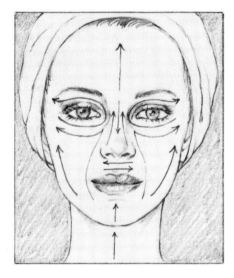

*1 A simple step-by-step massage can be followed like a simple cleansing action. The arrows show in which direction you should be working not only to cleanse your face with cotton wool but to continue massaging with fingers.*

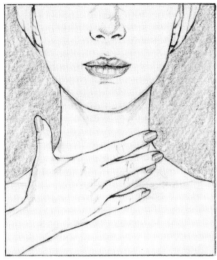

*2 **Neck** From left to right use firm overlapping strokes, and back again from right to left in at least eight movements.*

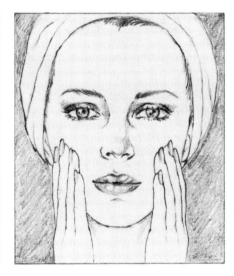

*3 **Contours** Start in two movements from both sides at centre of jaw moving under contour to cheekbone. Alternate hands with fingertips in a rhythmic motion. Then follow on in three movements up sides of the face to laughter lines and gently out under eyes.*

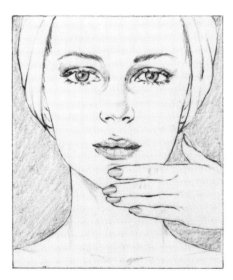

*4 **Lower contour.** Start in two movements across upper lip, left to right and back again. Then in four movements do vertical strokes up chin.*

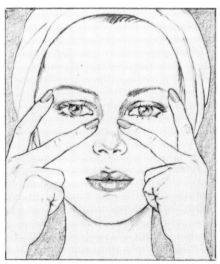

*5 **Forehead and eyes.** With both hands, use circular movements from outer corners of eyes, move under lower lashes, up and over lid, lifting at the end of the movement. Do not touch lashes. This should be done in two movements. Repeat, then return to centre of forehead.*

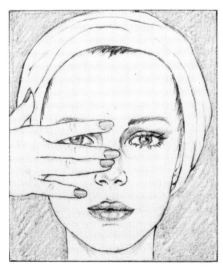

*6 **Nose.** Make three stroking movements down centre of nose; two movements in small upward strokes on left side of nose, and then right side of nose.*

# Behind the mask

The evolution of new, well researched formulae has led to the development of a new generation of face masks and packs which offer everything from lifting tiny facial lines to sloughing off dead surface skin cells (exfoliation).

Primarily designed to deep-cleanse, face masks are instant beauty treatments. Many masks also have toning, moisturizing, stimulating and exfoliating actions.

## Which mask for you?

There are different masks for different skin types – dry, greasy, normal, problem and sensitive. You may need to put a mask on just one section of your face, or even use two masks at once – a greasy-type one on your nose and forehead for example with a dry-type one on your cheeks. And, as your skin changes with the seasons, you may need to vary your masks according to the time of year.

**Cleansing masks** The most common type, principally for normal, combination and oily skins. They normally contain clay which absorbs impurities, removes blackheads and tightens the pores. They have a milk bleaching action to lighten the skin but also have a drying effect as they harden.

**Conditioning beauty masks** These act by gentle constriction of the skin during hardening to give a temporary tension. Blood vessels dilate in the deeper layers of the skin and fluid escapes resulting in a surface plumping effect. Fine lines temporarily disappear, the pores constrict and the face appears smoother.

**Peel-off masks** These are based on plastic, rubber or wax. They harden completely over the skin's surface, acting as a humectant – holding the moisture in and temporarily sealing the skin. When peeled off they remove dirt and dead cells. They accelerate the natural elimination of dead cells and generally firm up tiny facial lines. They're not really suitable for sensitive skins.

**Moisturizing or softening** This type of mask usually contains ingredients such as glycerine, gluci-

*A weekly treatment with a face mask is essential for good-looking skin, especially for those who live in pollution-laden towns.*

tol, and neutral amino-acids, which improve the skin's ability to retain moisture by attracting it, and by forming a barrier to slow down its loss from the skin.

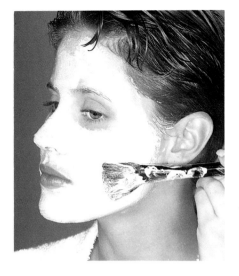

**Exfoliating masks** These are superficially formulated to remove dead surface cells, open blocked pores and remove excess blotchiness. Exfoliation is useful for more mature skins, since removing dead surface cells stimulates the formation of new ones. Chemical exfoliating masks *dissolve* dead surface cells while others exfoliate by physical

*You don't have to skip a treatment if you've forgotten to buy a mask – try some of the home-made recipes below. Whipped egg white (left) can be patted on or applied with a brush. Avocado (below) will improve a dry skin.*

abrasion. Some clay or mud-based masks contain camphor and warm on application. Apart from opening the pores, they're great for pepping up the circulation and can brighten sallow complexions.

**Cream beauty masks** These masks do not set hard and are ideal for sensitive or dry skin with a tendency to fine thread veins. They can be used frequently, as they don't exfoliate but simply refine the skin's texture. Apart from creamy formulas that wash off easily, they are available in mousse or soothing gel forms.

## Home recipes

If you have time you can always whip up your own face mask at home. Egg white tightens open pores and firms up a sagging skin. Whip up the egg white (you can add a little lemon juice) and pat across your face, avoiding eye area. Leave for 10 minutes.

If your skin is super-sensitive, try a gentle carrot mask. Grate the carrot, bind it with a little honey and pat on to the skin. (Carrot is packed with vitamin A – a wonderful skin food.) Avocado is perfect for dry skins. Mash avocado flesh with egg yolk and safflower oil or honey.

A winning mask for oily skin is made with tomato and lemon. Take one medium-sized tomato and mash it with the rind of half a lemon and a squeeze of lemon juice. Pat the mixture across the entire face, except for the eye area, and rinse off gently after 10 minutes with warm water.

Oatmeal is also used in many masks as it's a natural softener and whitener and, if used as oatmeal grains, an exfoliator. For a softening mask it's always best to add oatmeal after it's been soaked in warm water for 10 minutes.

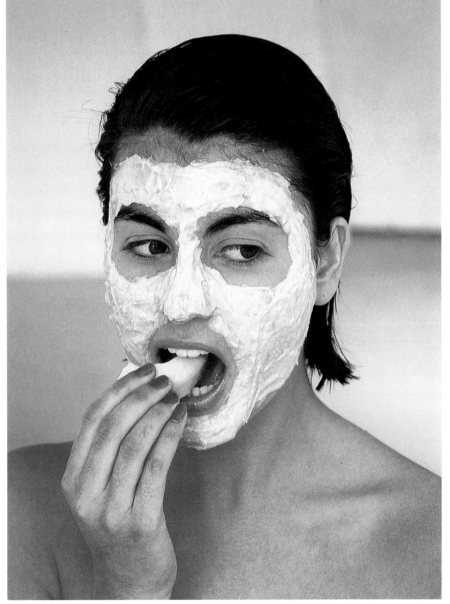

# All About Make-up

*Whatever your age, make-up will enhance your looks . . . and looking good is half the battle towards feeling good about yourself. Putting on your best face will give you confidence to face the world. The perfect make-up requires practice – and a little time. The steps shown on the next 12 pages take 15 minutes – time that some of you may feel you can't afford every day, while others – particularly those working in the public eye – may feel it's worth every second. But whatever you do, there are tips and tricks here that will give your make-up a longer-lasting, natural-looking polish. Whether you're just about to start using cosmetics or feel your old régime needs up-dating, we have some tips for you!*

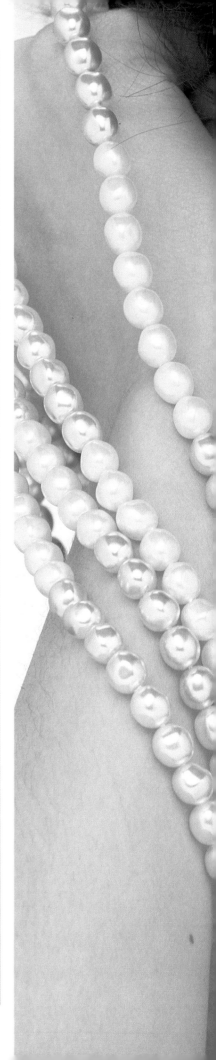

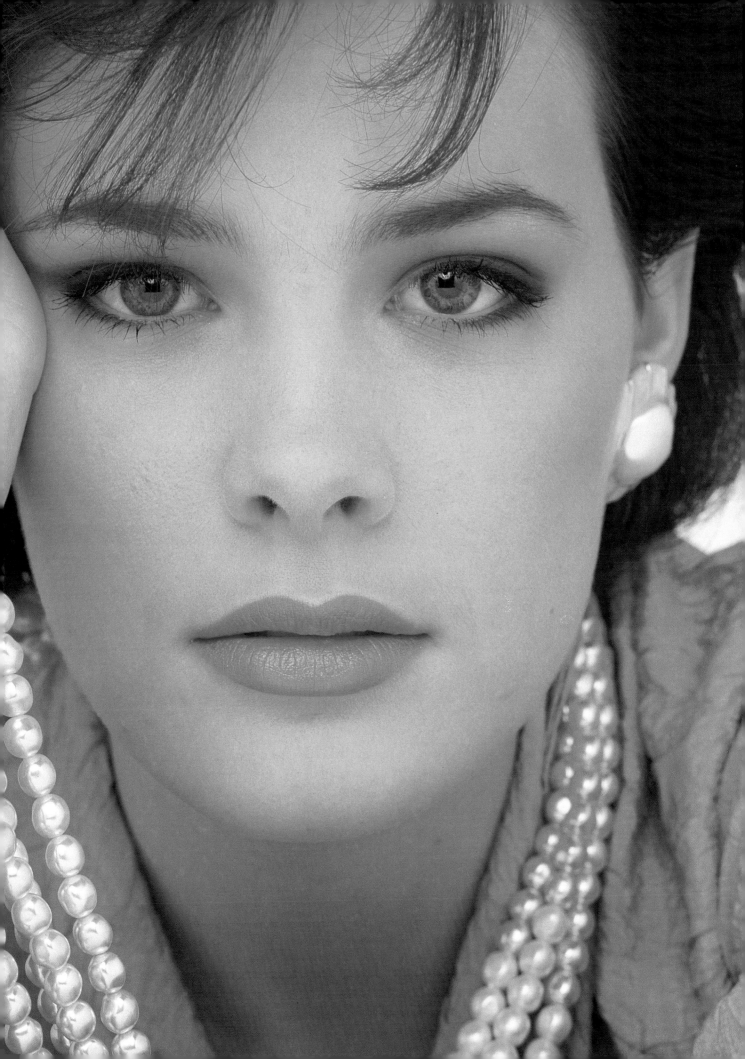

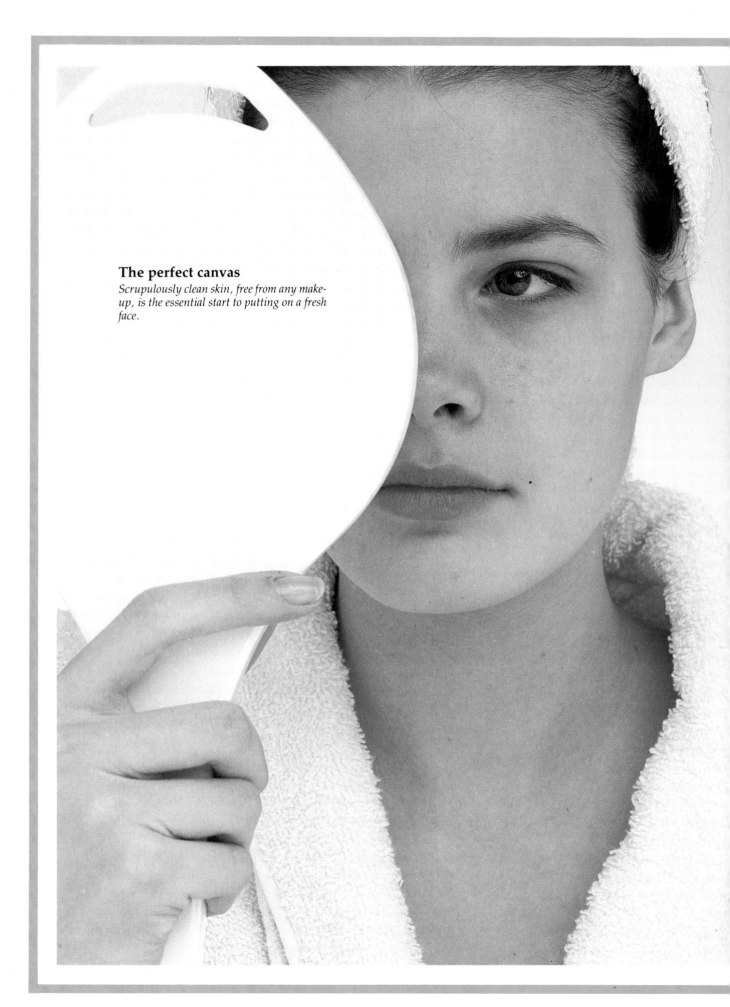

**The perfect canvas**
*Scrupulously clean skin, free from any make-up, is the essential start to putting on a fresh face.*

# A step-by-step guide to a perfect make-up

## Moisture must

Moisture creams or lotions not only keep skin smooth and supple but, when applied before foundation or base, they also create a barrier protection. Apply your moisturizer five minutes before smoothing over base. If you've been too liberal with your cream, blot excess moisture with a tissue.

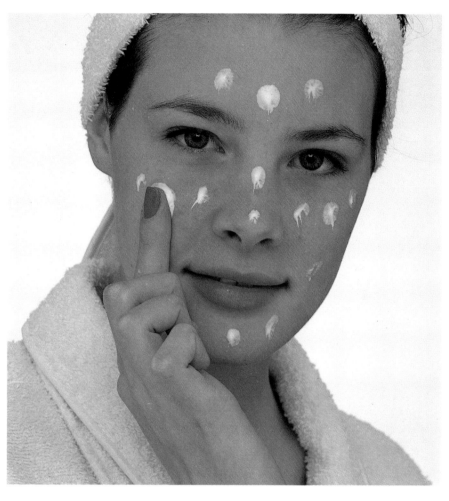

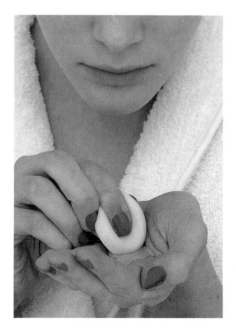

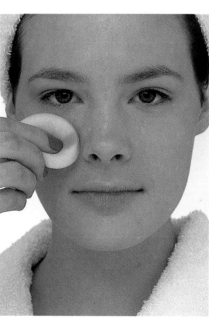

## Base tips

A damp sponge is essential if you want to smooth on foundation and ensure even coverage. It's best to squeeze your foundation into the palm of your hand since if the colour isn't quite right you can always mix two shades together.

Using the sponge, apply foundation from the centre of the face and work in outward sweeps; don't forget that you need to blend in under the chin or you'll see a demarcation line. Too much foundation under the eye area will emphasize wrinkles and crinkles. Blend the last trace of foundation in by lightly tapping over face with finger tips.

## Cover-ups

Very few of us have a spotless complexion or all-over, even skin tones so, after foundation has been applied, use a good camouflage stick like Elizabeth Arden's Erase. Do under eyes to take away dark circles; dot on cheeks for broken veins or high colouring; pinpoint nose area to hide open pores or simply cover up the odd spot.

Care should be taken around the eye area. The secret of good camouflage is to look down into the mirror so you can see exactly where the darker lines are and then apply. Blend in with a stipling action using ring finger.

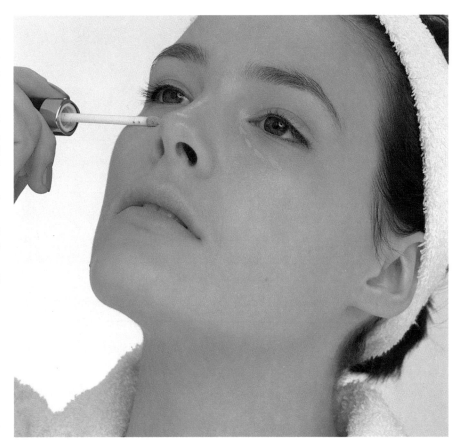

## Dust up

Now that you've got the perfect even colouring, keep it that way by using a translucent loose powder to seal in foundation. Roll a cotton-wool ball into powder and press onto skin – sparingly under eyes. You can be fairly generous with the powder to start with and then use a large bristle brush to sweep off the excess downwards so that fine facial hair isn't lifted up. If you still think you look a bit chalky, stroke lightly over face with fingertips.

There was a time when compact powder was frowned upon by top make-up artists because it didn't have the translucent quality of loose powder; it went on unevenly and left streaky marks. That era is firmly past. Pressed powders now glide over the skin like loose powder.

Powder is best used on top of your base make-up before applying blusher. It will keep your make-up in place for up to eight hours, so it's a must if you want your 'face' to last.

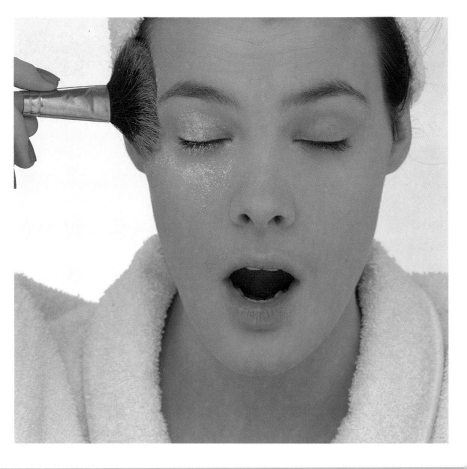

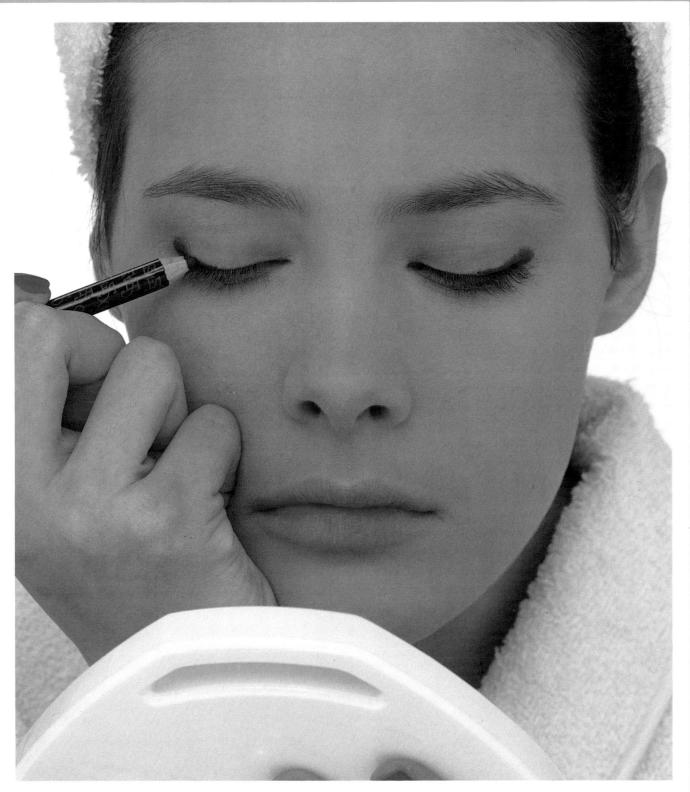

## Eye power

**Pencils** are great for giving shape to eyes and outlining where your colour should go. Always use a soft eye crayon or pencil which won't stretch the skin and can easily blend in with your powder or cream eye shadows. Choose your colour to suit your mood. On our model our make-up artist, **Bruce Hunter,** used a black crayon for a more dramatic outline but you can opt for a softer brown or grey. Take the pencil one-third of the way along the upper and lower lids as close to the lashes as possible. You can then use a cotton bud or damp brush to smudge the lines for a softer effect, working from outer to inner corners to avoid the old-fashioned 1960's winged effect. We then softened the pencil line by just using some brown shadow.

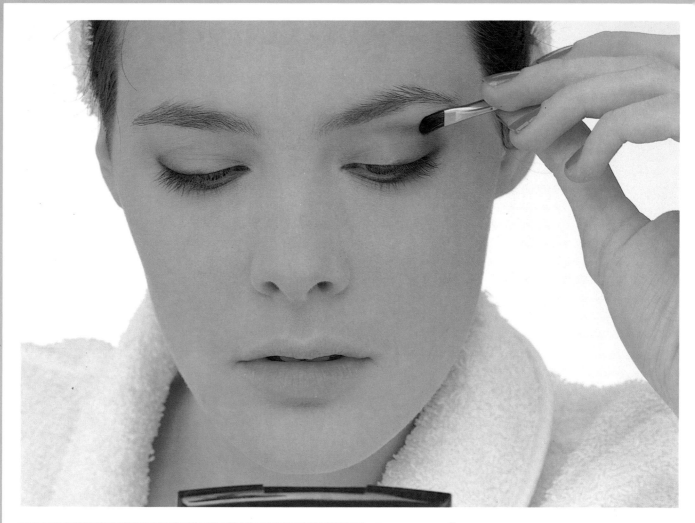

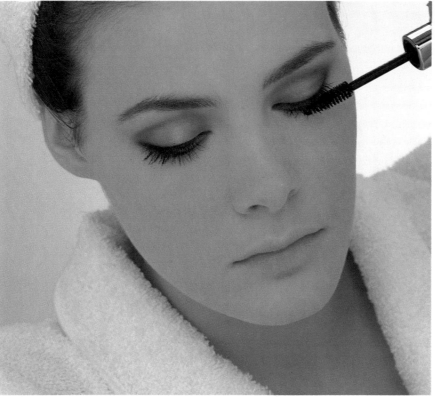

**Powder shadows** are more versatile than cream shadows and tend not to lie in the tiny crease lines. Always look straight into the mirror so you can see exactly where your socket line is. On our model we applied dark brown shadow halfway in socket line from middle to outer corner and then blended with a brush. We used pale brown shadow on the lid itself up to the socket line and then blended it into the darker brown. We used pale brown highlighter on centre of lid and above socket line.

**Mascara** gives eyes total balance. Do the bottom lashes first to avoid smudging. Do not apply more than two coats or lashes will look like clogged up spiders' legs. Let each coat dry first and then comb through. You can use eyelash curlers first to give lashes a lift.

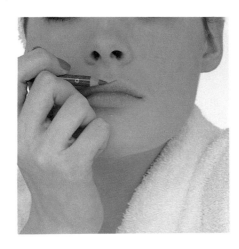

### Lip lines

**Lip liners** are good for correcting lip shapes – making lips look bigger or smaller. You can use a brush with a darker coloured lipstick or simply a lip pencil to outline lips. (Liner also stops lipstick from smudging.) Here we've emphasized our model's 'cupid's bow' shape to give the mouth extra definition.

**Lipstick** is always best applied with a brush but before doing this two-minute job, think about how you're going to get the staying power. Elizabeth Arden's Lip Fix cream, used before lipstick, stops the colour from running and smearing. Simply apply your base or foundation over lips or powder to build up a barrier. (Blotting out lips with base is also useful if you want to change their shape.)

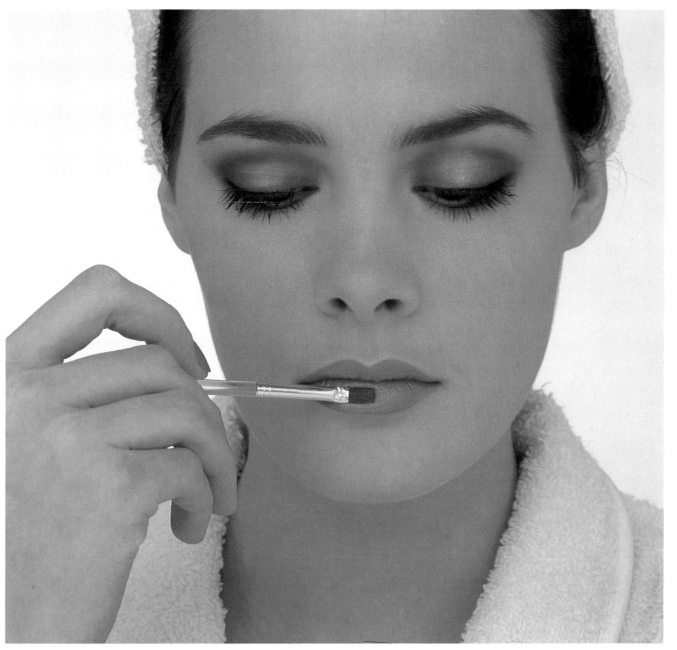

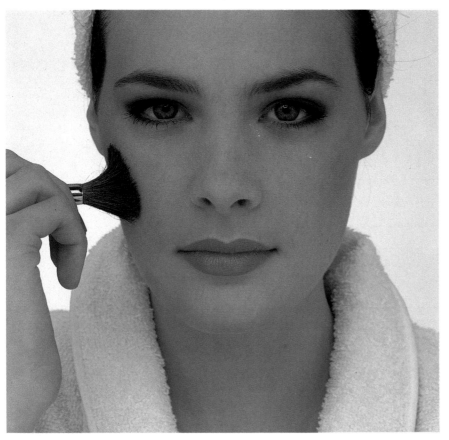

## Blush on

Powder blushers are easier to control than creamy ones since the excess can be brushed, rather than smeared off. Use a large powder blusher brush, dip into powder, shake off excess or blow or rub on back of hand before applying.

To find your cheekbones, put your thumb under your eye and straight down onto bone to find the curve. Never take blusher in further than half way under eye level. Using the brush, sweep on cheekbones and brush outwards to hairline. Soften with fingertips. The aim of blusher is to create a healthy and glowing look, not a sculptured one.

Blusher needn't be restricted to cheeks. It can be used under chin line to soften a long face and over eyelids for an extra lift. It can also be used lightly on sides of temples to give balance.

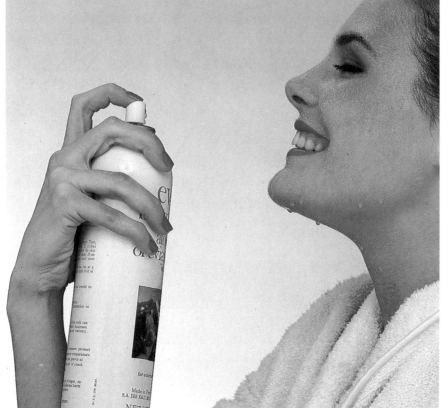

## Water fresh

A light spray of Evian (or equivalent) water can soon take the chalk-like look off freshly done make-up and give the skin a natural sheen. Apart from giving you an instant refresher, it can also help to set your foundation.

## The perfect finish

Chop and change with lip colours and blushers to match or contrast with your wardrobe. Experiment with eye shadows to match your mood rather than the colour of your eyes. It's up to you to make the most of yourself and create a confident image in your own style.

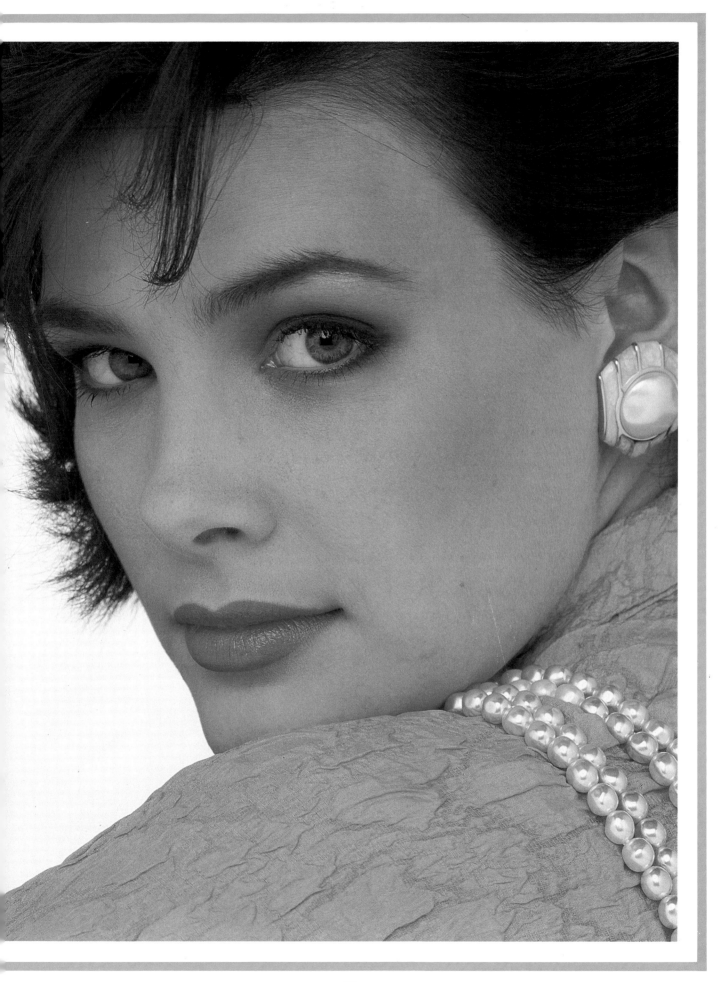

# Powder tips

● Choose a translucent powder to finish base; if you prefer a tinted powder, opt for a shade as close to your own skin tone as possible.

● Green powder has the power to take sallowness out of olive skins which have a tendency to look a little jaundiced at the end of summer.

● Green is also great on ruddy complexions which often fire up in fierce weather conditions. Just dust on a little green complexion powder to tone down any blotchiness or red colouring – then add your normal powder to tone all over.

● To thicken eyebrows, brush in a little powder and then use your eyebrow pencil to colour before brushing through to blend.

● For an evening effect, use loose powders with added shimmers to give a lustrous illusion.

● Don't confine your powder blushers to cheeks alone. Pink not only enlivens your cheeks but also brings a glow to temples and chin.

● If you prefer to use creamy eye shadows, give them staying power with a dusting of translucent powder so that the cream doesn't set in crease lines of lids.

● If you want your lip colour to last longer, apply base first, then powder, then apply your lipstick.

● If you have overdone the blusher you can tone down with translucent powder to take away the bright edges.

● To keep your powder fresh as the day you bought it, wash out all make-up brushes and powder puffs frequently.

# Lip tricks

Even if your lips aren't as lusciously shaped or perfectly painted as those in cover girl close-ups, with a little camouflage and top make-up artists' tips, you too can pout prettily.

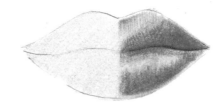

**1 To make your mouth look larger or smaller**
*Top: wear light, bright colours with added gloss to enlarge lips. Right: to trim down thick lips, wear darker, muted colours.*

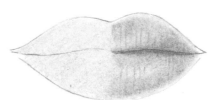

**2 To create fuller lips**
*Build up thin lips by applying a lip-liner pencil, a few shades darker than your lipstick, directly above your own natural lip line. Blend with a brush so there's no demarcation line.*

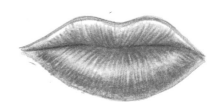

**3 To reduce full lips**
*Using a lip-line pencil just a few shaders darker than your lipstick, apply it just inside the lip line, making the mouth appear smaller. Blend again.*

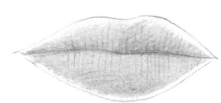

**4 To cheer up a droopy mouth**
*Lipstick can brighten up any face. If your lower lip is slightly droopy, outline it upwards with a pencil in a shade slightly darker than your lip colour. Draw attention to the upper lip by keeping the bottom lip colour darker than the top lip. Finish by dabbing gloss on the centre of the upper lip only.*

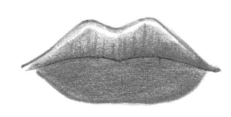

**5 To whiten teeth**
*If your teeth are less than perfectly white, choose a lipstick shade to camouflage. Pinks or reds with a slightly plum or mauve tint will make teeth look much whiter. Avoid browns and corals.*

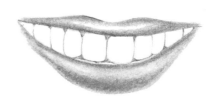

# Eye openers

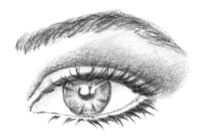

**1 To enlarge small eyes**
*Use a pale eye shadow nearest your lashes up to the crease line. Apply a dark, smoky colour in the crease. Repeat with a pale shadow (preferably with a sheen) over the crease and up to the browbone from the pupil diagonally out to the outer edge of brow. Blend the crease line so it merges with the highlighter. Line your eyes with a smoky liner close to all of top lashes but only half way under lower rim. Avoid inner rim liners unless you use white. Apply lots of mascara.*

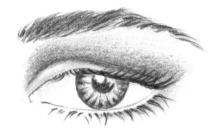

**2 To camouflage an overhanging upper lid**
*You could look sultry but if you want to correct an overhanging upper lid, use a dark colour in the crease line and continue it right up to the browbone. The dark colour should make the puffy lid recede a bit. Remember that light shows off and dark recedes. Use lots of mascara and a good make-up artist's tip is to apply a few individual false lashes at the outer corner to give 'lift' to the lid.*

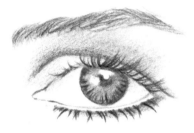

**3 To lift droopy eyelid corner**
*The secret of giving this outer eyelid corner a lift is to stop applying eye shadow and highlighters just before reaching the outer corner. Line under lower lashes with a dark kohl pencil and bring the line upwards at outer corner. Apply extra coats of mascara above the iris to draw attention to the centre of the eye rather than the outer corner.*

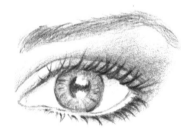

**4 To elongate round eyes**
*Make round eyes more almond-shaped by applying one shadow over the entire lid, starting above the inner iris and working diagonally up and outwards onto the browbone. Smudge the shadow around and under lower lashes on the outer corner only. Use mascara only on outer corners of eyes framing just the outer half of the eye.*

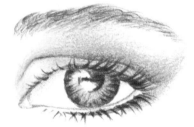

**5 To open up close-set eyes**
*Make sure you don't have any straggly brows in the centre of the brow line. Use a brow-bone highlighter from lash base to brow on the inner third of your lid (tear ducts upwards). Then use your eye shadow from base to brow bone, feathering it outwards slightly behind the outer edge of the eye both above and below. Use your eyeliner a third of the way from inner corner of both upper and lower lashes. Use mascara more on the outer two-thirds of upper and lower lashes.*

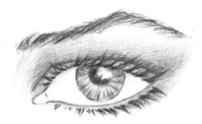

**6 To widen a narrow upper lid**
*Stick to just one medium-tone eyeshadow and extend it almost to the brow bone. You can use this same shadow to outline the outer third of the lower lid. Line the inner rim of the lower lid with a blue or mauve/lilac pencil to draw the focus away from your narrow upper lid. Use mascara but avoid curling lashes.*

## Lashes and brows

If your lashes are very fair, or you're going on holiday where water sports, rather than make-up, are your main concern, consider having your lashes tinted professionally.

Remember that lashes are hair, so treat them gently. When removing eye make-up each night, don't rub around the lash area. Instead, place a tissue beneath the bottom lashes and, closing each eye alternately, stroke an eye make-up remover pad gently down over top and lower lashes onto the tissue.

For thicker-looking lashes, apply loose powder before using mascara. On top lashes, apply first coat from topside of root to tip, second coat from underside of root to tip. Always allow a minute for mascara to dry between applications. Bottom lashes should normally only have one light coating at outer edges.

Always brush brows into shape after complete make-up. An old clean toothbrush does the job well – and removes any surplus base or powder.

If your brows are unruly, try brushing through a tiny dot of Vaseline or hair gel to keep them in shape.

If your brows are very fair, don't pencil them in with one continuous line. For a more natural look, pencil in tiny upward strokes in mid-brown or grey and then brush through for a softer effect. If your eyebrows are much darker than your hair colouring, they can be lightened professionally or you can do it yourself with careful use of facial hair bleaching products.

Eyebrows should be plucked – never shaved. Don't pluck into a thin line – merely tidy up stragglers across bridge of nose and from underside of brow.

*Well-defined brows draw attention to the eyes, when plucking don't overdo it – merely neaten up natural shape.*

To find out the right shaped brow for you, try this pencil test.

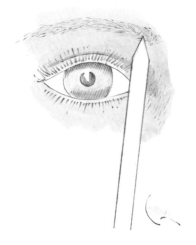

1 *Place a pencil along the side of your nose. The tip shows where the brow should begin.*

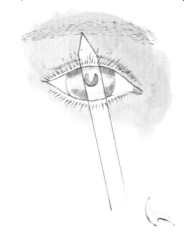

2 *Hold pencil at an angle with the tip passing across the centre of the pupil – this marks the highest point of the brow.*

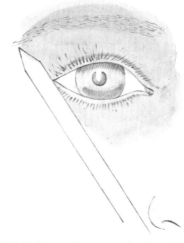

3 *Hold the pencil at an angle where the tip passes across the outer corner of eye – this is where the brow should end.*

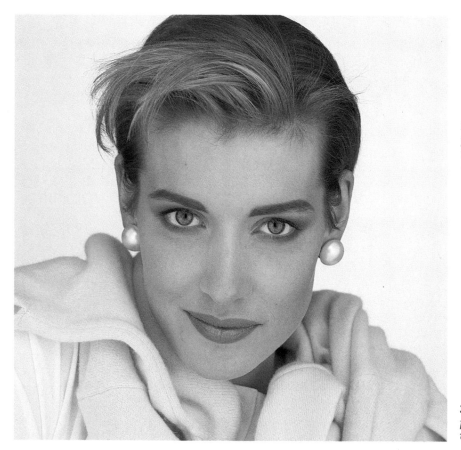

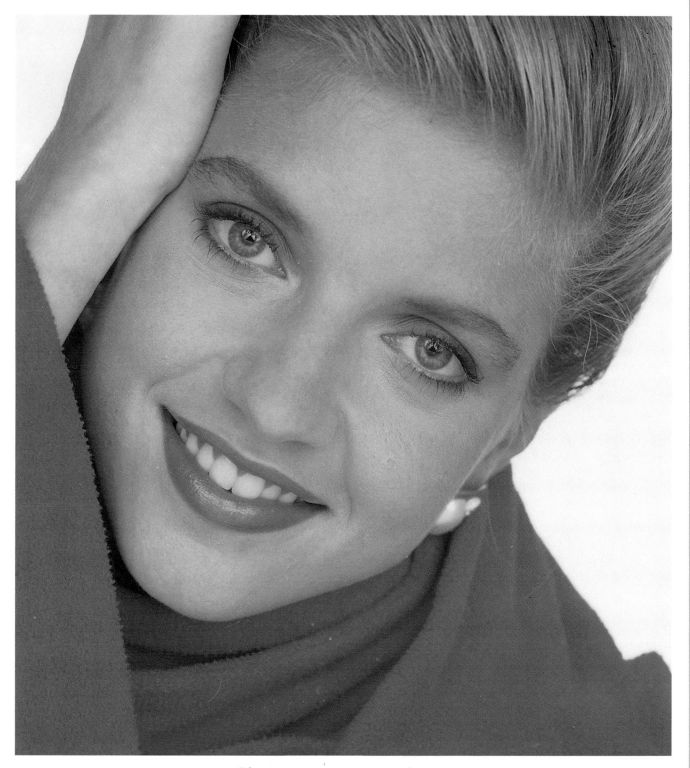

*Show your true colours*

Whether you're a redhead, blonde, brunette or have black hair, there's a colour range to suit your natural colouring, and the three pointers to your natural colouring are your hair colour, eye colour and skin tone.

**Fair skin**
Think of the Princess of Wales's complexion, and there you have the classic, dewy radiant look which instantly gives meaning to expressions like 'peaches and cream' and

'English rose'. Fair skin is associated with blonde/fair hair, light blue or green/grey eyes, and fair eyebrows, and is by far the most common skin type in Anglo-Saxons. In tip-top condition, a fair skin has the translucent quality of fine porcelain, but although much admired in youth, a fair skin is among the first to show its age.

This is mainly because it is susceptible to red spidery veins when exposed to extreme temperatures and, after 25, the skin will have a tendency to dryness, reacting badly to soap and water which will leave it feeling taut.

Younger skin can be cleansed with a mild non-alkaline soap like those in the milky and glycerine ranges, toned with a non-astringent toner, such as rosewater, and lightly moisturized.

Better protection is provided later on with a humectant cream (one that attracts moisture from the atmosphere). Lancôme's Bien Fait du Matin for dry/sensitive skin is a humectant and comes in three tinted shades.

**Base** Make the most of your peaches-and-cream complexion by using a thinner base/foundation. For a sheer, even colouring, choose a shade that is translucent.

**Blusher** If you are blonde, the pinks are for you. Don't be heavy-handed and choose colours close to your natural skin tone. Mousy blondes should look for warmer coral shades to brighten up their looks.

**Eye shadows** Subtlety is the key. Don't be influenced entirely by the colour of your eyes; lilacs and soft browns often complement green, blue or grey eyes beautifully but the rule is, if you blend softly, then you can wear practically any shade.

**Lips and nails** For blondes any shade of pink looks great, so do corals, apricot colours and brilliant, bold reds.

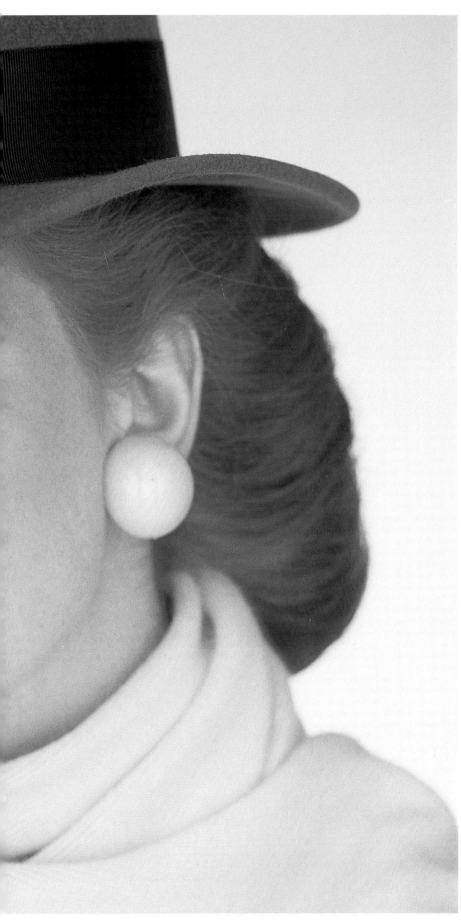

## Freckled skin

People with freckled skins usually have blue, green, grey or brown eyes, gorgeous auburn or Titian-coloured hair and a milky delicate complexion. Those of us who don't have them find freckles charming, but the freckle-skinned teenager usually hates them. Trying to cover them up or blot them out with skin-lightening creams doesn't really help the condition of your skin. They do fade with age but will reappear in the sun.

The appearance of freckles, usually over bridge of nose and scattered across cheeks, is caused by a lack of melanin (the body's own protective agent against the sun) in the skin. This makes freckled skin fragile, so at the first glimmer of sun, opt for a sunblock with high protection.

**Base** Don't try to cover your freckles with a ton of foundation. First apply a moisturizer with a green tint under an ivory tone foundation. This will take any redness out of your skin.

**Blusher** The terracotta shades are right for you, particularly if you have red hair. Pinks can be too overpowering.

**Eye shadows** Gold looks fabulous but always use it subtly, blending it with other colours from the terracotta spectrum. Greens with gold and lilac also look good. Always use lashings of mascara if you have fine, feathery eyelashes, and you may need to pencil in brows finely in a light brown eye pencil shade. If your lashes are fair you could invest in an eyelash tint which would save constantly applying mascara. They normally last between six to eight weeks.

**Lips and nails** Bronzes look brilliant and so do brown/reds. Avoid cerise, plum and true reds.

## Olive skin

A classic olive skin usually has a Mediterranean origin and at its best glows with good, healthy colour. Olive skin is honey-coloured with high cheek colouring and is associated with dark or black hair.

It does, however, pose a few problems in youth (spots, blemishes and an over-oily complexion) but the bonus is that it ages more slowly than other skins as its abundant natural oils continually lubricate the surface and prevent it from drying out. The pores are larger and the skin often shows an oily centre panel. It will settle down between the ages of 25 and 40 when it is at its best. Although olive skins tan faster than other skin types, it's still wise to deter the ageing process by using a sun filter cream. And you must use a lightweight moisturizer to keep skin supple and smooth: patch-treat oily areas with a mild astringent toner and, if you tend to suffer from blackheads and spots, a once-a-week mask is a boon as an intensive cleanser, ridding pores of impurities and skin of dead surface cells.

**Base** Choose a foundation which will not clog pores and, when carefully applied, will last for ages. Opt for a water-based foundation.

**Blusher** Highlight your natural colouring with bronze or peach colours. A powder shadow will last longer than a gel.

**Eyeshadows** You can wear the most dramatic colours and outline your eyes with pencils, kohl or eyeliner. Of course, no mature skin looks good made up with harsh colours but if you are under 35 you can afford to be daring.

**Lips and nails** Wear pillar-box red and carry on down through the red/brown spectrum. In summer, pink contrasts beautifully and looks stunning against a suntan.

## Black skin

In America, where the most comprehensive research has been done into black skin, there are at least 36 different shades, including those of Indian, African and Asian origins. Black skin at its best looks enviably free of lines. Teeth look whiter than white and eyes flash against their ebony background. But black skins can be fine and fragile and consequently need careful attention.

Pigmentation is often a problem; many black girls say their top lip is one shade darker than the bottom lip. The contraceptive pill may also cause light pigmentation of the skin.

Some colours can look slightly 'grey' or 'ashen' but can be brightened up if the top layer of dead surface cells is given a thorough exfoliation treatment, either with granule scrubs or a face mask.

The best news for black skins is Fashion Fair, a brand of make-up

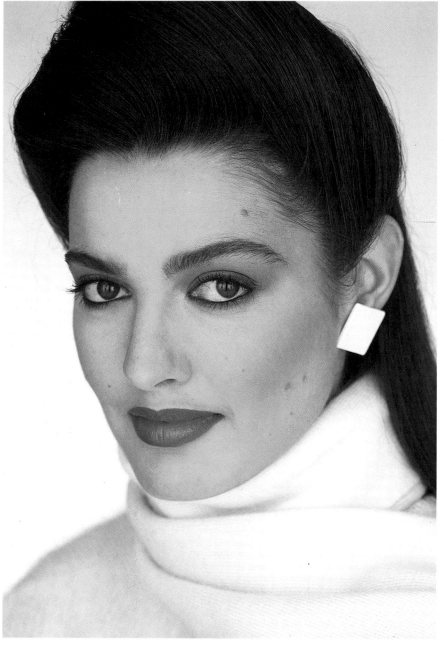

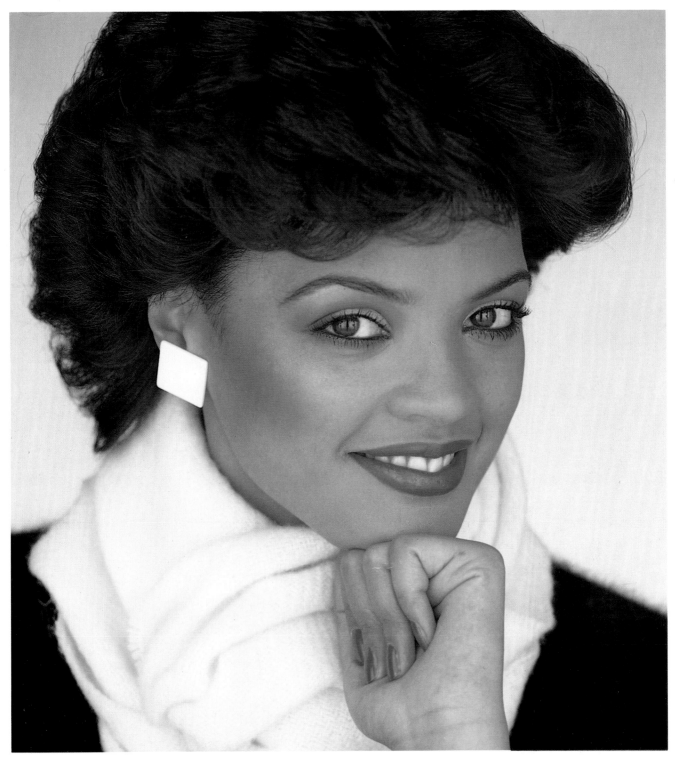

specially designed for dark skins. The collection also includes cleansers with facial shampoos for oily skin and special concentrates for dry skin.

**Base** Nearly every dark-skinned girl needs a concealer stick to blend out any pigmentation. Fashion Fair's Cover Stick comes in three shades.

For the base there are nine shades from light tan to chocolate. If the neck is one shade lighter than the face, choose a colour between the two.

**Blusher** Pinks through to plums are best for dark skins. Use a shade that will harmonize well with both your lips and nails.

**Eye shadows** Colours can be positive, strong and vibrant. Light and dark shades together will add depth and sparkle. Choose lilac, blue, turquoise, pink and copper.

**Lips and nails** Use Fashion Fair's Lip Balancer for a corrective lip stain. Keep lip, nail and cheek colours compatible.

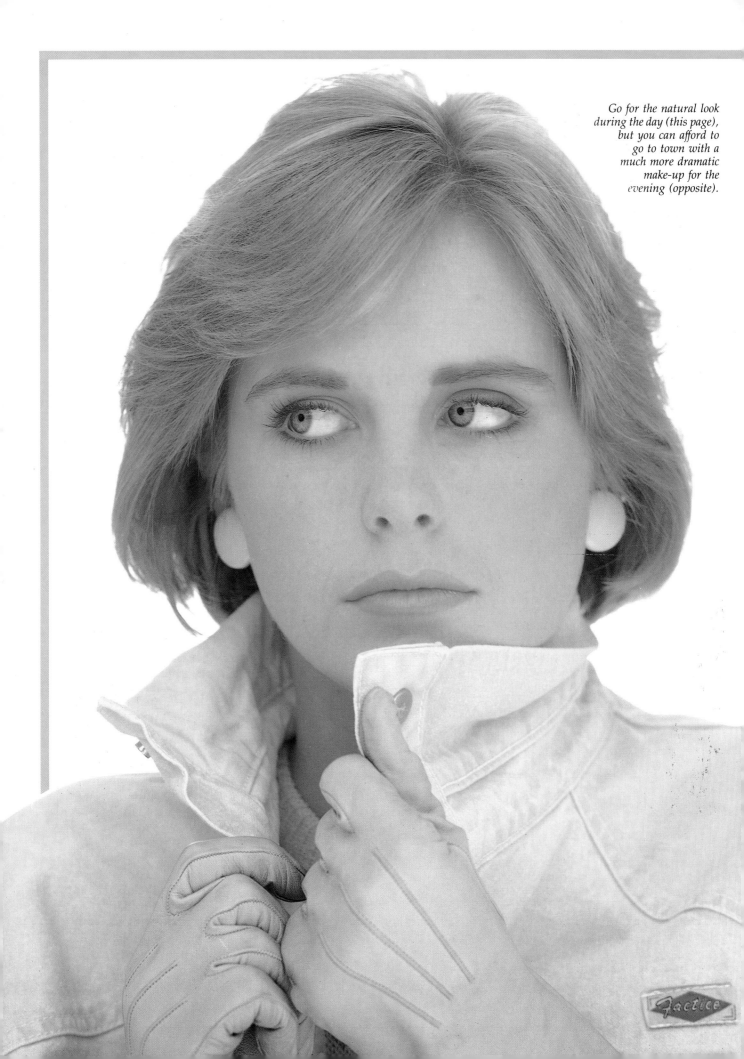

*Go for the natural look during the day (this page), but you can afford to go to town with a much more dramatic make-up for the evening (opposite).*

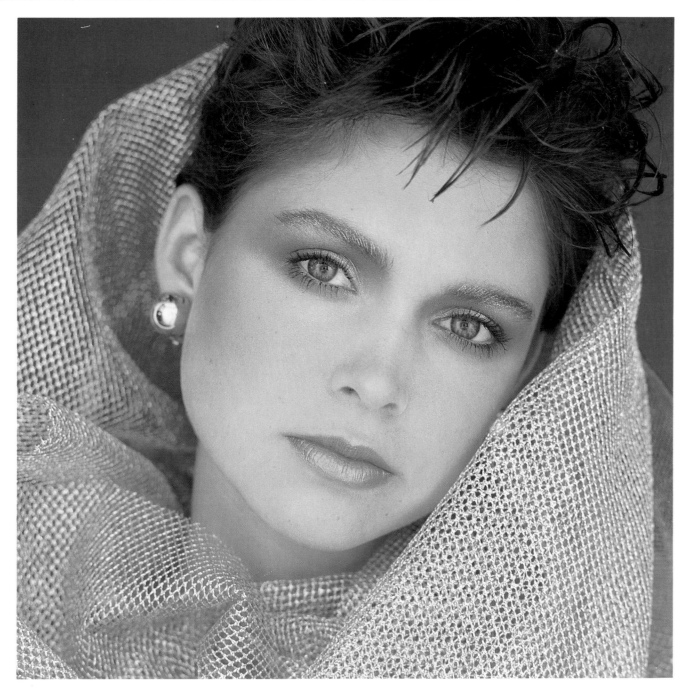

## Day face

The simplest of make-ups need only take a couple of minutes. Whatever your skin type, never skip on moisturizer and if your natural skin tone is pale or uneven, look for the products that combine moisturizers with a light tint. Then apply a coat of mascara. If your lips are thinnish, outline them in pencil and fill in with lipstick. If your mouth is generous, brush on a tinted lip gloss.

Apply a second coat of mascara. Use a dual purpose eye brush/comb to separate lashes and brush through brows. Finally, if you don't like a shiny look, use a translucent block powder and, if you need added colour, a slick of blusher.

## Evening face

You can create a really special basic make-up by adding gloss and glitter. For long-lasting lip colour, apply two coats – blotting in between – and then brush on gloss. Use a frosted highlighter shadow on lids – and opt for a face powder with speckles of gold or silver *or* a blusher with an iridescent sheen. (Don't go over the top and use both.) You can afford to be more dramatic with eye make-up at night – look for eye pencils in dark jewel shades or try midnight blue mascara instead of the usual black, grey or brown colours.

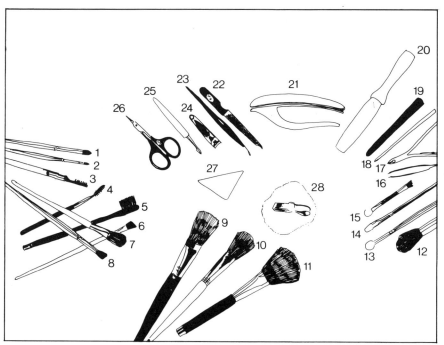

## Equipment that counts

There are so many handy up-to-the-minute beauty tools around to give you the perfect finish that you don't have to be a professional to do an expert job on your make-up and manicure. Here's a round-up of some of the best tools of the trade.

**1** Outline lips the professional way with a lip brush: it stops lipstick from smudging and smearing into fine crease lines around lips. After lining, fill in rest of lips with lipstick. Lip liners can also lip correct. Too full lips can be trimmed by using liner just *inside* the natural line and too thin lips can be made

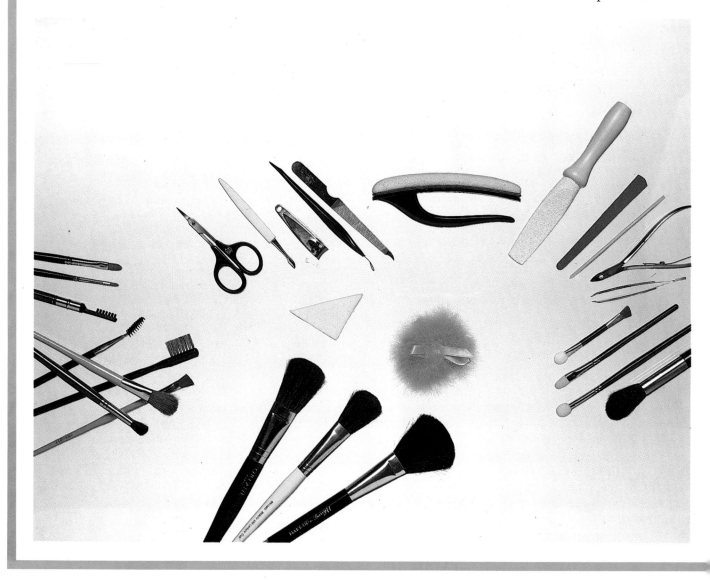

fuller by lining just above the natural line shape.

2 Eyeliner brushes are back but not necessarily to give you the black eye rimmer line of the Sixties. They can be used to line close to lashes with subtle smoky colours to change or enhance the shape of the eyes, or simply to contour a colour in the crease line before blending.

3 Brush up on your brows with a special stubbly brush or you could even use an old, clean toothbrush.

4 A curved mascara brush is handy for separating lashes before building them up with a second coat of mascara. Make sure they dry in between coats.

5 A wide bristly eyebrow brush cleans off excess powder or foundation and helps to shape up brows.

6 An angled eye-shadow brush is great for applying and blending shadows – particularly if you want to concentrate colour and 'wing' shadows to give an almond-up-shape effect.

7 Highlighter or blusher brushes should be light and easy to sweep across the cheekbones without leaving great splodges of colour. Sweep your highlighter just above the cheekbones where you apply your blusher, and blend outwards towards hairline.

8 A general blending eye-shadow brush can soften eye shadows and highlighters under the brow line so that they all blend in beautifully. It can also sweep off excess powder after colouring has been applied with a sponge-tipped applicator to give a more natural effect.

9 Wide, soft-haired brushes with loosely packed bristles give an even, light dusting of face powder. Use a translucent powder which doesn't alter the shade of your foundation or base. Dip brush in powder, shake off excess and brush from forehead *downwards* to chin to

avoid lifting up and accentuating tiny facial hairs.

10 Smaller brushes can be used for shading or contouring. Use a darker colour shadow stroked just under the cheekbones in the hollows of cheeks to slim down a round face. A small triangle dotted just under the chin and blended downward also helps to reduce a double chin.

11 Blusher brushes should be long-haired and fairly wide so you can sweep along cheekbones in one or two flicks. Always place blusher *on* your cheekbones just under the centre of eye, and brush outwards and upwards towards hairline.

12 Soft, thick, stubbly brushes are used to concentrate colour in one specific area before blending. They are good for contouring and shaping (placing powder slightly darker than your own skin tones) just under cheekbones, chin and forehead to camouflage various face shapes.

13 For smooth, even colour on eyelids use a round sponge applicator to spread powder evenly all over lids.

14 Use a contoured sponge applicator to eye shadow into crease lines before blending.

15 With a sponge and brush duo you can smooth on shadow with the sponge applicator at one end and sweep off excess powder with the brush at the other end.

16 Shape brows with tweezers, pulling out straggly hairs from the centre and hairs clinging to eye make-up underneath. To find out how to shape a natural line, see page 40.

17 These nippers are ideal for tidying hangnails. Never snip away at cuticles around the 'moonshape' of the nail. If they are badly ragged all round, seek the help of a professional manicurist.

18 Orange or manicure sticks are useful for cleaning under nails and pushing cuticles back. With cotton wool wrapped around the tips, they can also be used for smoothing over eye shadows.

19 A wooden double-sided emery board, with one rough and one smooth side, does a professional job of shaping and smoothing nails. Always file one-way from outer edge of nail into centre.

20 Tough, stubborn skin on heels and soles of feet can be smoothed away with a hard skin reducer – a contoured 'pumice'-style stone which can be used dry.

21 For really perfect nails, add that final sheen with a chamois leather buffer which not only polishes but also stimulates the nail-bed circulation and helps nail growth.

22 Stainless steel nail files are fine for emergency snags, and the hooked end is useful for cleaning under nails, but emery boards are far kinder to nail tips.

23 This cuticle trimmer has a pronged edge that neatly whisks off dead skin around sides of nails.

24 Rounded clippers trim down the toughest of nail lengths. Don't forget to shape and smooth nails with an emery board after clipping.

25 This small scraper is useful for cleaning under and around softened cuticles, but go gently.

26 If you've mastered the art of manicure (see pages 148 to 149), then you can expertly trim hangnails and cuticles with these slim cuticle scissors.

27 A small facial sponge is perfect for smoothing on foundation and base. If used damp, it will save on foundation and give an even spread.

28 Polish off the shine with powder applied with a soft, swansdown powder puff.

## The professional approach

Meet four of *Women's Own's* favourite make-up artists – and follow their tips to help give your looks a professional finish.

### Barbara Daly

Leading make-up artist and author of several beauty books, Barbara Daly had made up many top stars and was chosen by the Princess of Wales to create her wedding day make-up.

Barbara's flair for applying make-up is true artistry. 'Every face I make up I get excited about. Everyone has her own special feature: a terrific nose, lovely mouth or beautiful eyes. There are too many rules about what we should and shouldn't have. Confidence, making the most of your looks and enjoying life are the best beauty bonuses.'

Barbara believes that emphasizing eyes is an important confidence booster – 'I wouldn't ever be seen without my mascara and eye pencil! When doing a full eye make-up, it's important to use the correct brushes – and to experiment. A general rule is to keep the lighter colour to the inner corner of the eye and the darker to the outside. If you use eyeliner, apply with a fine, pointed, thin brush and take the colour as close to the lashes as possible. Avoid making hard black lines – dark brown or grey liner is more flattering.'

Brushes have been Barbara's tools

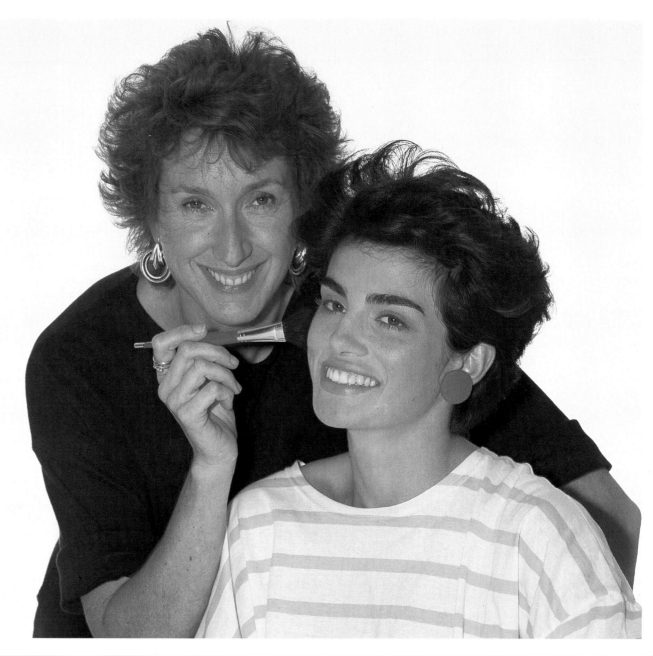

of the trade ever since she left Leeds College of Art in the Sixties. She believes there's a suitable brush or pencil for every make-up application. (Before the make-up companies flooded the market with coloured eye pencils, she improvised using artists' crayons!) 'If you use translucent powder, apply it with a loosely bristled, wide powder puff brush. Always brush off surplus powder in downward strokes to flatten tiny facial hairs,' is her tip. 'Use a round, stubbly brush for blusher. Dip it in, shake off excess, then dot the colour on cheekbones and blend upwards towards the hairline.'

Barbara believes that good skincare is vitally important for good looks. 'Choose products to suit your skin type and use them daily. It doesn't matter which system you opt for as long as you cleanse, tone and nourish faithfully. If you've cleansed your skin once and think it's enough – cleanse again. You'll be surprised at the grime that comes off. I'm equally fussy about clean hair – you can never rinse enough!'

## Maudie James

When she was just 16, Maudie James became a top international model – a career she followed for 14 years until, in 1980, she decided 'enough was enough' and became a make-up artist. 'It wasn't such a surprising decision,' says Maudie, whose clients include The Queen Mother, Princess Anne and Princess Alexandra. 'When I started modelling there were no make-up artists on a session – we did our own. I remember once going to Ethiopia with Norman Parkinson for *Vogue* – it was over 100°F and he wanted a 'tiger' look with elaborate eyes – and hair to match!'

These days when she's working, Maudie's own make-up is a lot simpler. 'I'm rather pale so I always wear foundation – it evens out my skin tone and helps to protect the skin against pollution. I also use

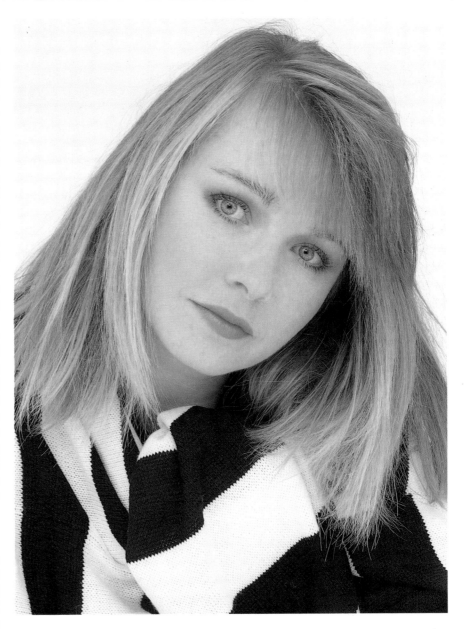

peach or pink powder on my eyelids and blusher on my cheeks – that's it.'

Her favourite products for the job include Lancôme's Maquisatin base and Estée Lauder's Country Fresh loose powder, 'because you can add and add it during the day and it doesn't go gloggy.' Her favourite eye products are Revlon's Charlie brown shadow ('You can use it for shading or add water and use it as a liner') and eyelash curlers. Maudie usually prefers neutral eye colours. 'When you're young you can try anything – but once a woman gets to 30 or so, neutral shades are much more flattering.'

Her tip if you want .to apply brightly coloured powder shadow: 'You should first apply lots of loose powder all around the eye, then apply the coloured shadow. If little wisps fall off, then you can just brush them off along with the base powder.' Maudie believes that everyone should have more than one shade of base. 'It's a mistake sticking to the same shade all year round. But I think the most common fault is using too much make-up. If you're making up for daytime, always do it in natural light by a window and, likewise, if you're making up for evening, do it by artificial light.'

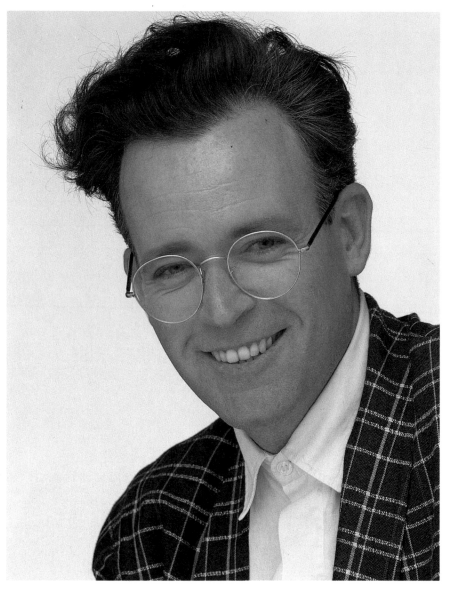

woman a wonderfully romantic look. Nigel explains: 'After moisturizer, I apply a deep cyclamen-coloured blusher to the cheek apples. I exaggerate it at first – it looks almost clown-like – then I buff the blusher with another clean brush, lightening it. I then apply the foundation *on top* of the blusher. After that, I take a tissue and peel it in half so it's wafer-thin, and press all over the face to 'blot' it. Third step is to dot a clean puff with powder, wrap the puff in a tissue and press all over the face. Remove surplus powder with a clean brush.

'Steam helps to give the skin a dewy look, so I'd recommend a bath before going on to finish the make-up on eyes and lips. It sounds complicated but I promise the end result is terrific.'

## Celia Hunter

Celia Hunter can't remember a time when she didn't want to be involved in make-up. 'But when I started out, you either worked in films or TV – there was no such thing as a freelance make-up artist. In fact, Barbara [Daly] and I were the first to step out on our own.'

Celia learned her basic training as an assistant at Max Factor. 'Then in 1967 I got a portfolio together and just went round magazines, saying 'Hey, why don't you use me?' Since then she's never stopped.

Celia has also worked on hundreds of commercials and produced four books. The most recent *Shades of Beauty*, is all about make-up for black skins. 'What surprised me when I first started working on the book was just how fine and delicate many black skins are – very sensitive to cold and wind. So proper skin care and daily moisturizing is a must. But a bonus black girls have is that they can wear bright colours for lips and eyes and heavily frosted shades which would look over the top on white women.'

Celia's own best beauty bonus is her thick mane of silver-white hair.

## Nigel Herbert

Australian Nigel Herbert was a commercial artist in Sydney who 'moonlighted' as a male model. 'I noticed there was a shortage of good make-up artists so I took a course that included stage and special effects – and suddenly I had a new career.' Since he moved to London in 1982 Nigel has worked non-stop.

His first lesson when he arrived? 'I had to throw away all the heavy bases I used to work with. I found the English skin was so good that it only needed the lightest of foundations.' Nigel's tip if you're shopping for a new base: 'When you're choosing in a department store, try it out on your neck – not your wrist. The colour on the neck and face should always match up – so apply a little, wander round the store for a while then go out into the daylight to see if it's subtle enough. Unless someone has very sallow skin where a pinkish tone base is best, the general rule is to opt for one with a yellow tone. If a concealer is necessary for shadows under the eyes or the occasional spot, I recommend Panstik. It's cheap, lasts for ages and does a good job.'

Nigel loves to do make-up for special occasions and this method (after a little practice) could give any

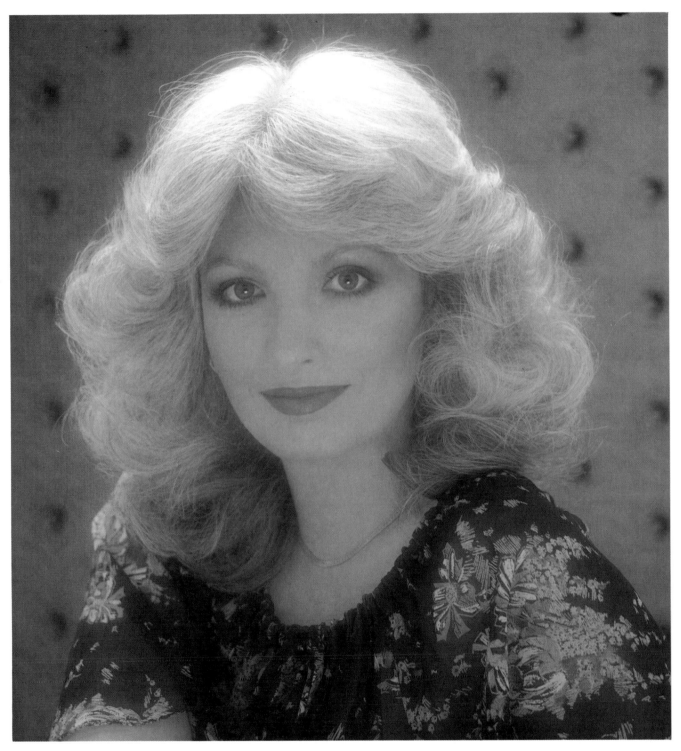

'It's naturally this colour. Both sets of grandparents went grey at a very early age – and my first silver hairs appeared when I was 11!' She has a professional semi-permanent colour with a hint of purply-blue by Wella applied every six weeks or so 'to make it look really clean. That may sound odd, but even a day spent in a studio where lots of people are smoking can give it a yellow tinge – and I find most mousses have the same effect.' For women who go grey at a slightly later age than she did, Celia recommends they check the shade of their make-up base. 'It's usually time to change to a lighter shade. But the rest of the make-up should be bright. Always use blusher – and even if pale lipsticks are the rage, stick to one with depth of colour. Eye shades, too, should have some density. I love brown shades but instead of a neutral tone, I use a rusty brown shadow that has more warmth. If you have silver hair, most bright shades of clothes look good. The only ones I avoid are the khaki and sludge shades.

# Getting into Great Shape

*Getting in great shape is really about keeping in shape. The varying physical and psychological phases of womanhood – adolescence, pregnancy, motherhood, menopause, old age – can gradually or dramatically change our bodies.*

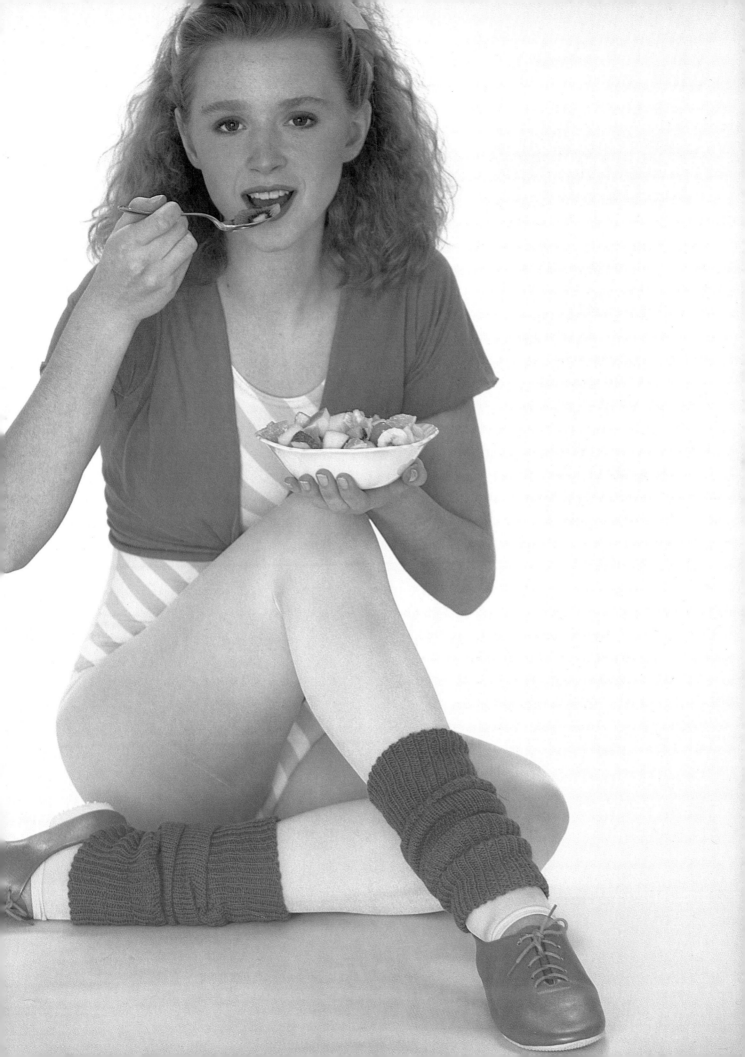

## Food for thought

You're fat because you eat too much has always been the simplest explanation for being overweight. You've tried every diet in the book, battled with the bulges for years and still the pounds have crept on. We can all lose weight in the short term by 'crash' dieting, but today's thinking, particularly from that august body, the Royal College of Physicians, says that crash dieting is dangerous and does little to help you adjust permanently to a more appropriate eating pattern for maintaining weight loss.

And it's not just how much we eat but what we eat. The fact that Britain has one of the highest rates of heart disease in the civilized world has prompted her Government to announce new laws to try to curb the fat content in our diet (fat contributes to heart disease; see opposite).

Diet alone cannot get your body in great shape. Exercise is also essential to keep your muscles in tone and improve your shape. If you are unable or unwilling to take up an aerobic exercise ie, one that puts continuous demands on your heart and lungs, making you puffed but not worn out) like swimming, jogging or a workout, you can try a 10 to 15 minute daily stretch routine to tone and condition your body (see pages 70 to 71).

Breaking old habits can be hard, but once you've set your mind to thinking *health*, you're one step towards a shapelier you.

## All about diets

Doctors and dieticians are now more likely to be 'social engineers' – helping us to look at the context of food as well as the content, so that we can work towards a healthier all-round lifestyle.

If you're among the one in three adults who is overweight, the

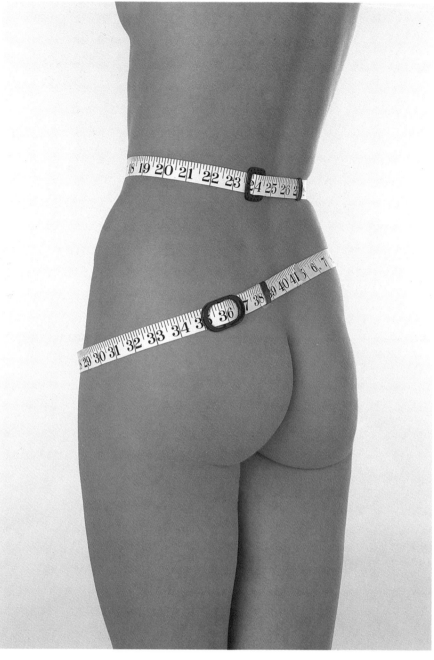

chances are you've tried to slim – and failed. Nine out of 10 people return to their original weight after dieting.

Why do we fail repeatedly? Quite simply, because when we've reached our target weights, we go back to our old eating habits. Those habits – as the NACNE (National Advisory Committee on Nutrition) and COMA (Committee on Medical Aspects of Food Policy) reports confirm – are the problem. Their reports reveal that the British diet is too high in fat (particularly sat-

*A sensible diet combined with regular exercise is the formula for a great shape. Follow our tips listed opposite.*

urated fat), sugar and salt and too low in fibre. Vegetable oils like margarine and cooling oils made from seeds contain unsaturated fats and are safer to use than animal fats.

**The fat problem**
In Britain a report by the Panel on Diet in Relation to Cardiovascular Disease (COMA 1984) recommends

that we reduce our fat intake by one-sixth and our consumption of saturated fats by one quarter.

At present we obtain more than 40 per cent of our energy from fat alone. Fat furs up the heart arteries and is one of several factors underlying heart conditions which kill one man in three, one woman in four; approximately 150,000 people a year. Smoking, being overweight, high blood pressure, lack of exercise, tension and inherited characteristics are also involved.

These risk factors are all interrelated – the pace of modern life can cause blood pressure to rise and tension and stress may be relieved by smoking. With pressure of work there is less time to take physical exercise or to eat balanced meals. Lack of exercise combined with a poor 'convenience'-style diet can result in people becoming overweight, which in turn increases their blood pressure. Fatty fried foods can cause their blood cholesterol level to rise and, in turn their blood pressure.

The influence of all these reports has resulted in tougher lines being taken in Britain, including the reccommendation that manufacturers should improve their food labelling – showing high, medium and low fat content, particularly in certain brands of sausages, and farmers will be asked to produce leaner sheep and cattle.

## What should you be eating?

The general formula is simple – increase your intake of fresh fruit and vegetables, potatoes and fibre (found in wholemeal breads, pasta and rice) and eat less sugar and starch. Cut down on milk, cheese, eggs, oily fish and red meats which contain hidden fats, and reduce your salt intake.

Any diet that promises a very rapid weight loss is likely to be unsuccessful in the long term. You'd lose more water than fat, put your health at risk and slow down your metabolism.

Crash diets of bananas and skimmed milk or the old favourite of grapefruit and boiled eggs may show quick results but are generally bad for your health and you will suddenly yearn for high-calorie sugary treats to compensate. Sugar may be a good energy booster for athletes who need glucose, but it is highly calorific and the calories are nutritionally 'empty'.

In general, a good diet is a varied one, well balanced, with a target of no fewer than 1,000 calories a day (see page 58), for a steady weight loss of one to two pounds a week. The slower the weight loss, the longer it is likely to stay off. (And don't forget to exercise, too.) Follow our weight chart overleaf and if you find you've more than 8lb/3·6kg to lose, try the Lifestyle Diet (on page 60). If you've less than half a stone to lose, here's a ten-point plan to lose those pounds healthily.

---

### Tips for wise eating

● **Buy low-fat dairy produce.** Choose skimmed milk, low-fat yogurt, low-fat spreads, Quark, curd and cottage cheeses. Use natural yogurt instead of cream in cooking. Limit eggs to three per person per week.

● **Eat more bread, pasta, potatoes.** These are filling but *not* fattening unless eaten with lots of fat or jams. Eat thick slices of wholemeal bread with a little low-fat spread, jacket or new potatoes with natural yogurt, parsley and chives.

● **Eat more fish.** It's low-fat, cheaper than meat and very nutritious.

● **Eat less meat and more vegetables.** Opt for poultry, rabbit, offal and less red meat. Buy lean cuts.

● **Eat more fresh fruit, vegetables and salad.** These are high in vitamins, minerals and fibre, and low in calories. Never overcook vegetables: place them in boiling water for no more than 10 minutes (potatoes excepted) and serve *al dente* or slightly crunchy, never soggy.

● **Eat less sugar.** The biggest culprits, apart from packed sugars, are sweets, and soft drinks. Cut out cakes, biscuits, puddings, jams. Choose cereals with no added sugar or unsweetened muesli.

● **Grill rather than fry food.** If you want to cook a casserole, trim fat off meat. With mince, it's best to boil quickly first with a minimum of water and then skim off the fat which has oozed out before adding sauces and popping in the oven. Use herbs rather than salt to flavour.

● **Read food labels.** Anything ending in 'ose' such as glucose or fructose, means sugar.

● **Choose fresh rather than processed foods.** Lots of manufactured foods have hidden fat, sugar or salt and preservative additives.

● **Start exercising.** Any aerobic exercise, done three times a week, for 20 minutes, will speed up your metabolic rate and help you to lose weight. Not everyone has the time to take up swimming, tennis, jogging or aerobic work-outs on a regular basis so at least make a daily 15-minute routine to shape up your body, (see pages 70 to 71).

# All about calories

Eating fewer calories than your body requires is the simple answer to losing weight – and there can be hardly anyone who hasn't at some time tried to lose weight on a calorie-controlled diet. In this age of technology all you need to tot up your daily calorie intake is a pocket calculator. With food manufacturers now being more label-conscious, we may even see calorific values being listed along with ingredients on packaged foods. Certain branded products are already showing these.

But there is more to losing weight than just counting calories: you must plan a well-balanced, nutritious diet (see page 60) which will give you all the daily requirements for health.

Why do you put on weight when you are sure you're not eating any more than normal? There are various explanations for this: one is that as you grow older, you need fewer calories per day. Another is your varying activities: the busy mum running around after a couple of toddlers is going to use up more energy than the secretary sitting at an office desk.

General statistics show that the average man needs around 2,500 to 3,000 calories a day (depending on occupation), whereas a woman requires between 1,700 and 2,500.

It's very difficult to work out your individual calorie requirements on a daily basis; instead, try calculating over a week to see if your input is more than your output.

For instance, if you are taking in 500 extra calories than your body requires, it will convert into 2oz/50g of fat so, to put on one pound in weight, you would have to consume around 4,000 extra calories. How long did it take you to put on that extra pound?

Remember that one large Mars bar has 453 calories and a Cornish pasty has around 417. So, if your daily intake is repeatedly 500 calories over, you gain a pound a week.

There's no reason why you shouldn't have a treat every day but not necessarily a bar of chocolate. Try something less calorific, like a ginger biscuit or a rich tea biscuit which contain around 50 calories each; then compensate by leaving out that slice of bread or extra potato for supper.

When you start counting calories you have to note everything you eat and drink and take into account that cooking can drastically alter the calorific values of raw food: 1oz/25g lard or cooking fat has 252 calories.

It's also worth noting that you'll probably lose more weight to begin with since the first energy stores you are depriving consist of starch which contains a lot of water. You'll lose this first along with a small amount of fat. After the first week you should get a good idea of your rate of weight loss in accordance with the amount of calories you are actually consuming.

## Weight chart for women without clothes

| Height | | Acceptable average | | Acceptable weight range | | Obese | |
|---|---|---|---|---|---|---|---|
| 4ft 10in | 1·47m | 7st 4lb | 46·0kg | 6st 8lb – 8st 7lb | 41·4kg – 53·6kg | 10st 3lb | 64·3kg |
| 4ft 11in | 1·50m | 7st 6lb | 46·8kg | 6st 10lb – 8st 10lb | 42·3kg – 55·0kg | 10st 6lb | 65·7kg |
| 5ft 0in | 1·52m | 7st 9lb | 48·2kg | 6st 12lb – 8st 13lb | 43·2kg – 56·3kg | 10st 10lb | 67·5kg |
| 5ft 1in | 1·55m | 7st 12lb | 49·5kg | 7st 1lb – 9st 5lb | 44·6kg – 59·0kg | 10st 12lb | 68·4kg |
| 5ft 2in | 1·57m | 8st 1lb | 51·0kg | 7st 4lb – 9st 5lb | 46·0kg – 59·0kg | 11st 0lb | 69·2kg |
| 5ft 3in | 1·60m | 8st 4lb | 52·0kg | 7st 5lb – 9st 8lb | 46·4kg – 60·3kg | 11st 7lb | 72·5kg |
| 5ft 4in | 1·63m | 8st 8lb | 54·0kg | 7st 10lb – 9st 12lb | 48·6kg – 62·1kg | 11st 12lb | 74·7kg |
| 5ft 5in | 1·65m | 8st 11lb | 55·4kg | 7st 13lb – 10st 2lb | 50·0kg – 64·0kg | 12st 2lb | 75·6kg |
| 5ft 6in | 1·68m | 9st 2lb | 57·6kg | 8st 2lb – 10st 6lb | 51·3kg – 65·7kg | 12st 7lb | 78·8kg |
| 5ft 7in | 1·70m | 9st 6lb | 59·4kg | 8st 6lb – 10st 10lb | 53·1kg – 67·5kg | 12st 12lb | 81·0kg |
| 5ft 8in | 1·73m | 9st 10lb | 61·2kg | 8st 10lb – 11st 0lb | 55·0kg – 69·2kg | 13st 3lb | 83·3kg |
| 5ft 9in | 1·75m | 10st 1lb | 63·5kg | 9st 0lb – 11st 4lb | 56·7kg – 71·1kg | 13st 8lb | 85·5kg |
| 5ft 10in | 1·78m | 10st 4lb | 65·0kg | 9st 4lb – 11st 9lb | 58·5kg – 73·4kg | 14st 0lb | 88·2kg |
| 5ft 11in | 1·80m | 10st 8lb | 66·6kg | 9st 8lb – 12st 0lb | 60·3kg – 75·6kg | 14st 6lb | 90·9kg |
| 6ft 0in | 1·83m | 10st 12lb | 68·4kg | 9st 12lb – 12st 5lb | 62·1kg – 77·9kg | 14st 12lb | 93·6kg |

The above height and weight chart shows the range within which your weight should stay and indicates when you are seriously overweight. Use it to set your target and remember that long-term dieting should result in a sensible weight loss of no more than 2 to 3lbs/1 to 1·5kg each week.

*If aerobics aren't for you – burn up calories with a sport from the list below.*

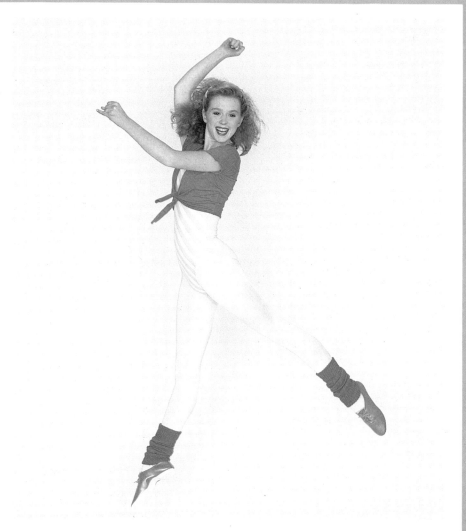

Most women can successfully lose weight on a diet consisting of around 1,200 to 1,500 calories a day, but may notice no weight loss the week before a period because of fluid retention. Don't worry, after menstruation, the weight loss will be greater.

The more gradual your weight loss, the more likely the pounds are to stay off. Never attempt to cut calories drastically to under 1,000 a day for any length of time. That said, it doesn't hurt the body to take in liquids only for a short time (see page 20).

Vary your foods and menus to keep your appetite stimulated (see our diets and recipes pages 61 to 69).

If you opt for a 1,500 calorie-controlled eating plan and find that you haven't lost weight after two weeks, then you are obviously using up less energy or you've forgotten to count in that walnut whip or slice of gateau. Reduce your calories by at least another day, cutting out a few items or simply making the portions smaller. Even if you think you are only losing ½lb/225g a week, don't despair; this is one of the most sensible weight drops as it enables skin to shrink naturally to cope with the slimmer you.

Nobody has to be a bore because of calorie counting. If you know you're going out for dinner then enjoy yourself and compensate for your indulgences throughout the week.

Remember that it takes longer to 'burn off' heavy meals eaten in the evening. Sleeping only burns up between 30 and 60 calories an hour.

Once you've established a gradual weight loss, give your body's metabolism a quick boost by varying your routine. If you find you come to a static point in your diet through no fault of your own, try taking more exercise. You should feel fitter and more energetic by now anyway.

Exercise tones the body, loosens the joints, stimulates the mind, gets the body's circulation going and shifts those stubborn fatty deposits.

### Burning up the calories

Here's a rough guide as to how some activities can burn up calories. (Bear in mind that a fatter, older person running for a bus is likely to use up more energy than a nimble teenager.)

Once you've achieved your target weight for height, age and build, you'll be surprised to find that you can eat and drink more without putting on weight (providing you continue to exercise) because you'll be feeling fitter, healthier, younger and more alive – not having to stock up on extra fuel simply to carry all that excess weight around.

| Activity | Calories per hour |
|---|---|
| Bowling | 200 – 300 |
| Cycling (15 mph) | 650 or more |
| Dancing | 200 (more for disco dancing) |
| Gardening | 200 – 300 |
| Golf | 300 or more |
| Housework (general) | 150 |
| Ironing | 250 |
| Jogging (under 5 mph) | 500 or more |
| Rowing | 1,000 or more |
| Sex | 250 – 1,000 |
| Skating | 300 – 500 |
| Soccer | 500 – 600 |
| Squash | 600 – 700 |
| Swimming | 300 – 600 |
| Tennis | 500 or more |
| Walking briskly | about 350 |

## The lifestyle diet

You can lose your fat for ever with a healthy eating plan involving less fat, less sugar, less salt and more fibre. Our 1,500 calories-a-day lifestyle diet combined with exercise (see page 70) will soon bring about a slimmer, fitter you.

### How to start

Our 31-day eating plan, based on between 1,300 and 1,500 calories a day, not only helps you to lose weight but suggests mouthwatering recipes to take the boredom out of dieting.

Every day, allow yourself ½ pint/ 300 ml milk, in addition to milk shown in the diet, for drinks. If you prefer your main meal at midday, swap the menus round.

All bread in the diet is wholemeal. Buy or make your own (see recipe page 67). The dough doubles as a pizza base. Some supermarkets sell frozen wholemeal pizza bases. We also suggest a recipe for muesli, or buy ready-made, choosing a brand with little or no added sugar (check ingredients on packet). Where we say 'buttered' on toast, use a margarine high in polyunsaturates or a low-fat spread (see recipe for home-made spread page 67) and spread it thinly.

All meat weights are for uncooked meat except where stated. Use a minimum of salt. Cut down first at the table, then in cooking. Gradually you should lose your taste for it.

Weekday lunches are designed to be portable to accommodate those who work away from home. You'll need a lidded, plastic bowl for salads and a wide-necked flask for soup. If you have a freezer, make up soups, bread, pizzas, lasagne, savoury corn pie and banana crunch slices in one go and freeze in portions or whole if you have lots of hungry bodies around to eat up what's left. The banana crunch

slices will keep fresh for up to 10 days in an airtight tin.

Saturday evening meals are special. Have them at home, entertain with them or choose them in a restaurant.

Very strict diets are doomed to fail – most aren't flexible enough. So use your common-sense. If you're out one evening and fancy a drink, have one, but cut the equivalent calories from your pudding. A glass of wine averages 80 calories, half a pint of lager 80, a gin and tonic 90, dry sherry 70.

If you haven't reached your target weight at the end of your 31 days, you can repeat the diet. It's safe to do so indefinitely.

If you are on target, or don't wish to go on slimming, forget calorie counting but keep your new good habits and gradually increase bread and potatoes until your weight stabilizes. Not only will this help you to maintain your figure, it will safeguard your health.

IMPORTANT: if you have a medical problem or are worried about your health, consult your doctor before beginning this diet and exercise programme.

*A nourishing breakfast like this is essential when dieting to keep energy levels high.*

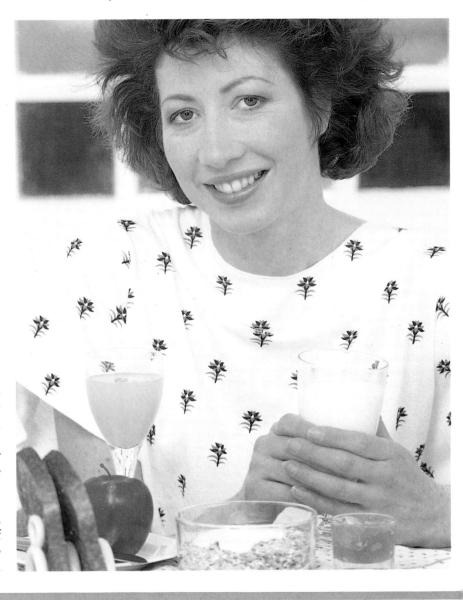

| Day | Breakfast | Midday meal | Supper |
|-----|-----------|-------------|--------|
| | **Week 1** *For dishes marked with an * see recipes pages 67 to 69* | | |
| **1** | 2 Shredded Wheat or 3 Weetabix with 5 fl oz/150 ml skimmed milk Slice buttered wholemeal toast* | 8 oz/225 g slice melon 1 hot pizza* Mixed salad* | 2 fl oz/3 tablespoons glass dry sherry 2 stuffed courgettes* 1 baked apple stuffed with teaspoon honey, pinch ground cloves |
| | **350 calories** | **422 calories** | **598 calories** |
| **2** | 8 oz/225 g slice melon 2 oz/50 g muesli* with 5 fl oz/150 ml low-fat yogurt | 4 oz/100 g chicken piece, baked 5 oz/150 g jacket potato 4 oz/100 g green beans 1 serving apple and walnut crumble* | 1 serving bean soup Slice wholemeal bread* 1 medium pear |
| | **315 calories** | **621 calories** | **427 calories** |
| **3** | 2 Shredded Wheat or 3 Weetabix with 5 fl oz/150 ml skimmed milk Slice buttered wholemeal toast* | Cheese salad (2 oz/50 g Edam, cubed, 1 tomato, shredded lettuce, ½ green pepper, few slices cucumber) 1 wholemeal roll* 1 tablespoon lemon dressing* 4 oz/100 g grapes | Cottage pie (4 oz/100 g lean minced beef or minced beef and soya, ½ onion, 5 oz/150 g mashed potato, 1 tablespoon tomato purée, pepper) 4 oz/100 g frozen peas 1 banana crunch slice |
| | **350 calories** | **435 calories** | **502 calories** |
| **4** | ½ grapefruit 3 oz/75 g kipper fillet, grilled Slice buttered wholemeal bread* | 1 serving vegetable soup* Salad sandwich made with 2 slices wholemeal bread* and mixed salad* 1 apple | 1 serving spinach lasagne* 5 fl oz/150 ml glass red wine 1 pear in 5 fl oz/150 ml red wine, baked below lasagne for 20 mins, served with 2 tablespoons low-fat natural yogurt |
| | **332 calories** | **459 calories** | **614 calories** |
| **5** | 2 oz/50 g muesli* with 5 fl oz/150 ml skimmed milk 1 medium banana | Tuna and tomato sandwich, with 2 slices wholemeal bread*, 3½ oz/90 g can drained tuna in brine and 1 tomato 1 medium apple | 1 serving savoury corn pie* 5 oz/150 g baked potato with 1 tablespoon low-fat natural yogurt Green salad* 1 pear |
| | **353 calories** | **444 calories** | **633 calories** |
| **6** | Porridge made with 1½ oz/40 g rolled oats, 5 fl oz/150 ml liquid (½ skimmed milk, ½ water) and 2 teaspoons honey Juice of 2 large oranges | Brown rice salad (½ 7·9 oz/220 g can kidney beans, 1 tomato, 1 oz/25 g brown rice, cooked, ½ onion, parsley, 2 tablespoon sprouting beans, 4 olives, lemon dressing*) | 4 oz/100 g liver and 1 slice back bacon sautéed in juice of 1 orange 4 oz/100 g mashed potato 4 oz/100 g frozen peas 4 oz/100 g carrots 4 oz/100 g grapes |
| | **324 calories** | **448 calories** | **592 calories** |
| **7** | 1 large apple and 4 oz/100 g grapes chopped into 5 fl oz/150 ml low-fat natural yogurt Slice wholemeal buttered toast* | 1 serving vegetable soup* 1 hard-boiled egg 2 crispbreads 1 banana crunch slice* | 6 oz/175 g mackerel, grilled 1 tomato, grilled 6 oz/175 g potatoes, boiled 4 oz/100 g cabbage 5 fl oz/150 ml glass dry wine |
| | **335 calories** | **425 calories** | **613 calories** |

| Day | Breakfast | Midday meal | Supper |
|---|---|---|---|
| **Week 2** *For dishes marked with an * see recipes pages 67 to 69* | | | |
| **8** | 1 grapefruit<br>1 lean rasher bacon, grilled<br>2 tomatoes, grilled<br>1 buttered wholemeal roll*<br><br>**322 calories** | 1 serving vegetable soup*<br>2oz/50g cottage cheese on 2 large grilled mushrooms<br>Slice buttered wholemeal toast*<br><br>**343 calories** | ½oz/15g dry roasted peanuts<br>2 glasses dry sherry<br>4oz/100g sirloin minute steak, lightly grilled, with green salad*<br>1 large baked potato with yogurt<br>8oz/225g slice melon<br>**666 calories** |
| **9** | 1½oz/40g bran flakes with 5fl oz/150ml skimmed milk<br>2 tomatoes, grilled, on slice buttered wholemeal toast*<br><br>**341 calories** | Hot pot (4oz/100g lean braising steak, 1oz/25g dried prunes, 3floz/4½ tablespoons brown ale, herbs, parsley, 4oz/50g potatoes) served with 4oz/100g green beans<br>Baked pear split and filled with 2oz/50g stewed apricots, 2 teaspoons honey<br>½pint/300ml beer to drink<br>**499 calories** | 1 Big Mac *or* Wimpy *or* restaurant pizza *or* 2 pieces Kentucky fried chicken and coleslaw *or* 1 doner kebab<br>Piece fresh fruit, such as a pear or apple<br><br><br><br>**Average 530 calories** |
| **10** | Porridge made with 1½oz/40g rolled oats, 5floz/150g liquid (½ skimmed milk, ½ water) and 2 teaspoons honey<br>Slice wholemeal toast* spread with small mashed banana<br><br>**358 calories** | Beansprout and date salad (3 tablespoons beansprouts, 1 chopped apple, 1oz/25g dates, ½oz/15g walnuts, stick celery and 1 orange)<br>Lemon dressing*<br>1 wholemeal roll*<br><br>**433 calories** | Portion 4oz/100g chicken, grilled<br>2oz/50g rice cooked with ½ chopped onion in chicken stock<br>3oz/75g broccoli<br>5floz/150ml glass dry white wine<br>Apple (5oz/100g) stewed with 4oz/100g blackberries with 5floz/150ml low-fat natural yogurt<br>**515 calories** |
| **11** | 1oz/25g muesli* with 1 chopped apple and 5floz/150g skimmed milk<br>Slice buttered wholemeal toast and Marmite<br><br>**355 calories** | 1 serving vegetable soup*<br>1 serving cold pizza*<br><br><br><br>**459 calories** | Chilli con carne (½ 7·9oz/220g can red kidney beans, 4oz/100g minced beef, 8oz/225g can tomatoes, 1-2 cloves garlic, crushed)<br>Fresh fruit salad*<br>**592 calories** |
| **12** | 2 Shredded Wheat or 3 Weetabix with 5floz/150ml skimmed milk<br>4oz/100g mushrooms cooked in dash lemon juice on slice buttered wholemeal toast*<br><br>**366 calories** | 1 serving bean soup*<br>1 wholemeal roll*<br>1 apple<br><br><br>**403 calories** | Cauliflower cheese (6oz/175g cauliflower, sauce: 5floz/150ml skimmed milk, ½oz/15g polyunsaturated margarine, ½oz/15g flour, 1oz/25g Tendale cheddar, grated)<br>1 banana crunch slice*<br>**584 calories** |

| | Week 2 *For dishes marked with an * see recipes pages 67 to 69* | | |
|---|---|---|---|
| **Day** | **Breakfast** | **Midday meal** | **Supper** |
| **13** | 5 dried prunes, soaked overnight in water to cover<br>1 egg, boiled<br>1 buttered wholemeal roll*<br><br>**350 calories** | Potato salad (1 large potato, cooked and chopped, parsley, 2 spring onions, chopped, 4 olives, 1 tablespoon French dressing*)<br>4oz/100g low-fat natural cottage cheese<br>8oz/225g slice melon<br>**424 calories** | Liver casserole (4oz/100g liver braised with 1 onion, 4oz/100g carrots, 6oz/175g potatoes, 8oz/225g can tomatoes, pinch oregano)<br>Fresh fruit salad*<br>2 tablespoons natural low-fat yogurt<br>**582 calories** |
| **14** | 1½oz/40g muesli* with 5floz/150ml skimmed milk<br>Slice buttered wholemeal toast*<br><br><br>**347 calories** | Liver sausage sandwich (2 slices buttered wholemeal bread*, cucumber, 1oz/25g liver sausage)<br>1 large orange<br><br>**447 calories** | 1 serving vegetable soup*<br>4oz/100g frozen cod steak grilled with ½oz/15g polyunsaturated margarine and served with sliced lemon<br>4oz/100g frozen peas<br>4oz/100g green beans<br>4oz/100g boiled potatoes<br>5floz/150ml glass white wine<br>**563 calories** |

| | Week 3 *For dishes marked with an * see recipes pages 67 to 69* | | |
|---|---|---|---|
| **Day** | **Breakfast** | **Midday meal** | **Supper** |
| **15** | 2 Shredded Wheat or 3 Weetabix with 5floz/150ml skimmed milk<br>Slice buttered wholemeal toast*<br><br><br>**350 calories** | 1 slice hot savoury corn pie*<br>Green or mixed salad*<br><br><br>**482 calories** | Salmon loaf*<br>2 tomatoes, sliced<br>2oz/50g each potatoes and onion, thinly sliced, baked in 5floz/150ml chicken stock for 30 minutes at Mark 6, 400 deg F, 200 deg C<br>5floz/150ml glass wine<br>Stewed apricots (soak 5 dried overnight in little water and simmer until tender, sweetened with a sweetener) topped with 5floz/150ml low-fat natural yogurt<br>**573 calories** |
| **16** | 1oz/25g muesli* with cored and sliced apple and 5floz/150ml skimmed milk<br>Slice buttered wholemeal toast* and yeast extract spread<br><br>**355 calories** | 4oz/100g grilled lamb cutlet coated in ½ beaten egg and breadcrumbs<br>2 tomatoes, grilled<br>4oz/100g boiled potatoes<br>5floz/150ml glass red wine<br>Rice pudding (2 level tablespoons pudding rice cooked with ½ pint/300ml skimmed milk, dash nutmeg, 2 teaspoons honey)<br>**571 calories** | Salmon salad sandwich (2 slices buttered wholemeal bread*, 1½oz/40g canned salmon, green or mixed salad*)<br>1 large orange<br><br><br>**446 calories** |

**Week 3** *For dishes marked with an * see recipes pages 67 to 69*

| Day | Breakfast | Midday meal | Supper |
|-----|-----------|-------------|--------|
| **17** | 1 pear and 4oz/100g grapes in 5floz/150ml low-fat yogurt Slice buttered wholemeal toast* with 1 teaspoon honey **324 calories** | 1 serving bean soup* 2 crispbreads 1oz/25g liver sausage and 4 radishes **433 calories** | 1 hot pizza* Green or mixed salad* 1 banana crunch slice* **580 calories** |
| **18** | 5 prunes, soaked overnight 2 Shredded Wheat or 3 Weetabix with 5floz/150ml skimmed milk 1 buttered crispbread with 1 level teaspoons honey **333 calories** | Sardine sandwich (2 slices wholemeal bread*, 4½oz/120g can sardines in tomato sauce) 4oz/100g grapes **440 calories** | 1 corn on the cob Macaroni cheese (2oz/50g macaroni, cheese sauce as for cauliflower cheese on 12th day) Green or mixed salad* 1 orange **582 calories** |
| **19** | 5oz/150g can baked beans on sliced buttered wholemeal toast* Juice of 2 large oranges **340 calories** | 1 serving vegetable soup* 1 rollmop herring Green or mixed salad* 1 buttered wholemeal roll* 1 pear **429 calories** | 4oz/100g pork fillet and 1 tomato, grilled 4oz/100g courgettes, sliced and steamed with ½oz/15g polyunsaturated margarine 4oz/100g boiled potatoes 1 banana crunch slice* **555 calories** |
| **20** | 2oz/50g muesli* with 1 cored and chopped apple and 5floz/150ml skimmed milk **330 calories** | 1 serving bean soup* 1 wholemeal roll* 4oz/100g grapes **467 calories** | 6oz/175g mackerel, grilled 4oz/100g boiled potatoes 4oz/100g green beans 6oz/175g rhubarb, stewed with a sweetener and topped with 3 tablespoons natural yogurt **542 calories** |
| **21** | Porridge made as for 10th day Slice buttered wholemeal toast* and marmalade **358 calories** | Egg bap (1 buttered wholemeal roll* 1 mashed hard-boiled egg and 1 tomato) 1 banana crunch slice* **470 calories** | 1 serving spinach lasagne* Green or mixed salad* Fresh fruit salad* with 5floz/150ml low-fat natural yogurt **568 calories** |

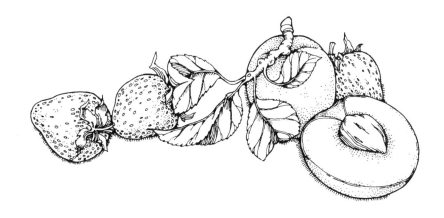

**Week 4** *For dishes marked with an * see recipes pages 67 to 69*

| Day | Breakfast | Midday meal | Supper |
|---|---|---|---|
| 22 | ½ grapefruit<br>1½oz/40g bran flakes with 5floz/150ml skimmed milk<br>Slice buttered wholemeal toast*<br><br>**343 calories** | 5oz/150g can baked beans on 2 slices buttered wholemeal toast* topped with 1 poached egg<br><br>**460 calories** | 5½oz/165g trout baked in foil with strips of carrots and celery (2oz/50g each) and served with lemon<br>4oz/100g boiled potatoes<br>4oz/100g frozen peas<br>Bread and butter pudding*<br>5floz/150ml glass wine*<br>**568 calories** |
| 23 | 5 dried prunes, soaked overnight<br>2 Shredded Wheat or 3 Weetabix with 5floz/150ml skimmed milk<br>1 buttered crispbread and 1 level teaspoon honey<br><br>**333 calories** | Tandoori chicken (6oz/175g chicken breast, marinated in 3oz/75g low-fat natural yogurt mixed with ½-1 tablespoon tandoori powder, then grilled)<br>2oz/100g boiled brown rice<br>1 tablespoon mango chutney<br>½ pint/300ml beer to drink<br>Grilled fruit kebab (about 2oz/50g each of apple, orange and banana)<br>**535 calories** | 1 slice hot savoury corn pie*<br><br><br><br>**447 calories** |
| 24 | 1oz/25g muesli* with 1 chopped and cored apple and 5floz/150ml skimmed milk<br>Slice buttered wholemeal toast* and yeast extract spread<br><br>**355 calories** | Beansprout and date salad made as for 10th day<br>1 tablespoon lemon dressing*<br>1 wholemeal roll*<br><br>**433 calories** | 3½oz/90g ham steak, 1 tomato, grilled<br>4oz/100g broccoli<br>4oz/100g boiled potatoes<br>Slice buttered wholemeal bread*<br>1 banana crunch slice*<br>**545 calories** |
| 25 | Porridge made with 1½oz/40g oats and 5floz/150ml liquid (½ skimmed milk, ½ water) and served with 2 teaspoons honey<br>Juice of 2 large oranges<br><br>**324 calories** | 1 serving bean soup*<br>1 buttered wholemeal roll*<br>4oz/100g grapes<br><br>**467 calories** | Cheese omelette (2 eggs, 1oz/25g Tendale cheddar cheese, grated, and ½oz/15g polyunsaturated margarine)<br>Green or mixed salad*<br>1 tablespoon French dressing*<br>1 banana and 1oz/25g dried dates chopped into 2½floz/4 tablespoons natural low-fat yogurt<br>**615 calories** |
| 26 | 2 Shredded Wheat or 3 Weetabix with 5floz/150g skimmed milk<br>Slice buttered wholemeal toast*<br><br>**350 calories** | 1 cold pizza*<br>Green or mixed salad*<br>1 pear<br><br>**431 calories** | Spaghetti bolognese (1 onion, ½oz/15g polyunsaturated margarine, 4oz/100g lean minced beef, 8oz/50g can tomatoes, 2oz/50g mushrooms, herbs)<br>3oz/75g wholemeal pasta<br>5floz/150ml glass red wine<br>1 apple<br>**596 calories** |

| Day | Breakfast | Midday meal | Supper |
|-----|-----------|-------------|--------|
| | **Week 4** *For dishes marked with an * see recipes pages 67 to 69* | | |
| 27 | 1½oz/40g muesli* with 5floz/150ml skimmed milk 2oz/50g mushrooms cooked in lemon juice on slice buttered wholemeal toast* 

355 calories | 1 serving vegetable soup* 1 hard-boiled egg 2 crispbreads 1 banana crunch slice* 

425 calories | Cheese jacket potato (1 large baked potato split and sprinkled with 2oz/50g grated Tendale cheddar cheese) Green salad* 1 tablespoon French dressing* 1 wholemeal roll* 1 pear baked as for 4th day 553 calories |
| 28 | 5floz/150ml carton low-fat yogurt with 1 large apple, chopped, and 4oz/100g grapes Slice buttered wholemeal toast* 

335 calories | 1 slice cold savoury corn pie* 

447 calories | Stuffed tomatoes (2 large tomatoes stuffed with 1oz/25g cooked brown rice, 3½oz/90g can tuna in brine, drained, ½ green pepper, juice of 1 lemon, parsley) 1 serving apple and walnut crumble* and 2 tablespoons yogurt 623 calories |
| 29 | 1½oz/40g bran flakes with 5floz/150ml skimmed milk 2 tomatoes, grilled, on slice buttered wholemeal toast* 

341 calories | Hot pasta and cockles (2oz/50g wholemeal pasta, boiled and drained, with 4oz/100g cockles, rinsed thoroughly, 8oz/225g can tomatoes, 1 chopped onion, 1-2 cloves garlic, crushed, heated together and poured on pasta) Green salad* 1 orange 

448 calories | 1 serving vegetable soup* Slice wholemeal bread* Lamb kebab (4oz/100g piece loin of lamb grilled with 1 green pepper in chunks) Ratatouille (3 tomatoes, ½ green pepper, 1 onion, 2 courgettes) Gooseberry fool (1¼floz/2 tablespoons yogurt, 1 beaten egg white, 4oz/100g puréed gooseberries with a sweetener) 5floz/150ml glass wine 625 calories |
| 30 | ½ grapefruit 1 boiled egg 1 buttered wholemeal roll* 1 teaspoon honey 

331 calories | 4oz/100g lean roast turkey 4oz/100g baked potato 4oz/100g swede 4oz/100g cabbage 1 large banana baked in juice of 1 orange and 1 teaspoon honey, and served with 3 tablespoons low-fat yogurt 576 calories | 1 serving vegetable soup* Turkey sandwich (2 slices buttered wholemeal bread*, 2oz/50g lean turkey, green or mixed salad*) 

489 calories |
| 31 | 1½oz/40g muesli* with 5floz/150ml skimmed milk Slice buttered wholemeal toast* 

347 calories | Potato salad (1 large potato, boiled and diced, parsley, 4 spring onions, chopped, 4 olives, 1 tablespoon French dressing*) 4oz/100g carton low-fat cottage cheese 1 orange 448 calories | 4oz/100g piece haddock, grilled 4oz/100g leeks, boiled 1 wholemeal roll* 1 serving apple and walnut crumble* 

612 calories |

# The recipes

## Wholemeal bread

Makes 4 × 1 lb loaves or 48 rolls or 12 pizza bases (4-5 in round); total calories 1,049

2 tablespoons soya oil
1 lb/450 g Wheatmeal flour
1 lb/450 g strong flour
1 lb/450 g Granary flour
1 teaspoon salt (optional)
pinch sugar
2 oz/50 g fresh or 1 oz/25 g dried yeast
1½ pints/900 ml warm water

Rub oil into warmed flours and salt. Activate yeast by creaming fresh yeast with sugar or mixing dried yeast with sugar and ¼ pint/150 ml of the water. Leave until frothy. Pour yeast liquid and remaining water into flour. Add a little extra liquid if required to make a soft, but not sticky, dough. Knead well for 5 minutes or until firm and elastic. Leave to rise (prove) in a warm place loosely covered with cling film or light greased polythene bag to prevent drying out. Grease and flour loaf tins or baking tray. When dough is double in size and spongy, knock back to original size and knead on a floured surface for 3-4 minutes. Cut into four for loaves, 12 for pizzas or 48 for rolls. Place in tins, or shape into rolls on a baking tray, or for pizzas roll into 4-5 in/10-13 cm rounds. Leave, covered, in a warm place until double in size and spongy. Bake at Mark 8, 450 deg F, 230 deg C for 30-35 minutes until golden brown. Remove tin. If loaf sounds hollow when tapped, loaf is cooked. Cool on wire rack.

## Low fat spread

Cut down your calorie and saturated fat intake by making your own spread for use in sandwiches and on vegetables. The healthiest one is made by whipping together 2 oz/50 g of a margarine high in polyunsaturates with 2 tablespoons water or water and skimmed milk. Store in fridge. Butter-lovers might prefer a 50/50 butter/soya oil mixture. Slowly whip together and store in fridge.

## Muesli

Serves 9; total calories 1,634

6 oz/175 g rolled oats
2 oz/50 g bran
1 oz/25 g barley or rye flakes
1 oz/25 g brown sugar or clear honey
2 oz/50 g raisins
1 oz/25 g sultanas
2 oz/50 g nuts, walnuts, hazelnuts or almonds, chopped
2 oz/50 g dried apples, chopped finely
2 oz/50 g dried dates, chopped finely
1 oz/25 g dried apricots, chopped finely

Mix all ingredients together and store in airtight container. Serve with cold or hot skimmed milk.

## Vegetable soup

Serves 12; 109 calories per serving

chicken carcass, skin and giblets
3-4 carrots
1 turnip
1 large onion
2-3 sticks celery
1 bay leaf
1 large sprig parsley
1 sprig rosemary
1 sprig thyme
6-8 peppercorns
2 quarts/2·25 litres water
6 oz/175 g macaroni
4 small potatoes, peeled and chopped

First make stock: wash chicken carcass in cold water. Prepare and clean giblets; discard any fat from skin. Put carcass in a large saucepan. Peel and chop vegetables and add to pan with herbs and peppercorns. Cover with water. Bring slowly to boil, and skim off scum when it rises. Cover and simmer very gently for 1 hour for a quick stock, 2 hours for a strong stock. For a more concentrated stock, leave off lid so that stock reduces during cooking. Strain, reserving vegetables, cool quickly and then remove fat by passing pieces of absorbent paper across the surface of the stock. To finish soup, add pasta and potatoes. Bring to boil, cook for 20-30 minutes, then add reserved vegetables.

## Bean soup

Serves 6; 223 calories per serving

4 oz/100 g dried cannellini beans
4 oz/100 g dried haricot beans
2 tablespoons polyunsaturated oil
1 onion, peeled and chopped
1 carrot, peeled and chopped
2¾ pints/1·5 litres good beef stock
1½ oz/40 g pearl barley
⅓ teaspoon dry mustard
2 tablespoons fresh parsley, chopped
2 oz/50 g green or yellow split peas
2 oz/50 g lentils
freshly ground black pepper

Soak beans overnight in water to cover. Drain. Heat oil and fry onion and carrot gently until soft. Add soaked beans, stock, pearl barley, mustard and parsley. Bring to boil, reduce heat and cover pan. Simmer for 45 mins. Add split peas and lentils, cover and simmer for further 40 mins. Season to taste with pepper.

## French dressing

Makes 5 fl oz/150 ml total calories, 754

2 tablespoons white wine vinegar or lemon juice
6 tablespoons soya oil
¼ teaspoon teaspoon dry mustard
sugar substitute (optional)
¼ teaspoon salt (optional)

Place vinegar or lemon juice, oil, mustard, sugar and salt in a screw-top jar. Shake well before serving. To add variety add 1 peeled and crushed garlic clove or 2 tablespoons finely chopped onion; or curry powder to taste.

## Lemon dressing

Makes 2¼ fl oz/4 tablespoons; total calories, 38

2¼ fl oz/4 tablespoons natural low-fat yogurt
2 teaspoons lemon juice
zest of ½ lemon
pepper to taste

Mix ingredients together in a screw-top jar. Shake well before serving.

## Sprouting seeds

Sprouting seeds are a simple, economical and soil-less way of providing a selection of fresh vegetables throughout the year. Choose from *mung bean,* giving the crisp, juicy Chinese beansprout; the *soya bean,* larger than the mung and more beany in flavour; the *aduki bean,* slow-growing, red-skinned, small and sweet; *whole brown or green lentils* which give a sweet peppery shoot (red split lentils don't sprout); *mustard seed,* tiny black seeds that grow rapidly to give hot, spicy sprouts; *fenugreek,* a large seed that grows in 4-5 days and is mildy curry flavoured; *tiny mint seeds,* even more tasty if you add a little extra mint; *wheat sprouts,* sweet and nutty, but choose only organically grown grain with no trace of pesticides.

Most health food and continental grocery shops stock a good selection of seeds.

*To sprout:* wash old jam jars well; cut a piece of J-cloth or fine cotton to cover top and hang 1-2in/3-5cm down sides of jars. Wash seeds and pick out grit and any broken seeds. Place 2-3 table-spoons seeds in each jar and cover with material, held in place with a rubber band. Fill with warm water and soak overnight in a warm place. Next morning, drain well and rinse seeds through cloth. Repeat rinsing 2 or 3 times a day for 3-6 days, depending on seed (5-8 days in a colder room), until sprouts are about 1½in/4cm long. The seeds can be grown in the dark or light. Those grown in the dark are pale cream coloured, while those grown in the light are streaked with green. Sprouts not rinsed or drained thoroughly develop musty stale flavours and those grown for too long tend to get tough and stringy.

*Keeping sprouts:* once sprouts have reached desired length, keep them wrapped in polythene in the fridge for up to a week. When freezing, they are best combined in a dish as they tend to lose their crispiness once thawed. Freeze for up to six weeks.

*Growing goodness:* most beans and pulses are rich in protein and once they start to sprout they become rich in vitamins too. The vitamin C content is nearly as high as in citrus fruit, and they are a good source of B vitamins. After 4 days of keeping, the nutritional value drops. Cooking destroys much of the nutritional value, so ideally, eat them raw. If you cook them, do so in the minimum of water – and save cooking liquid for stocks and gravies.

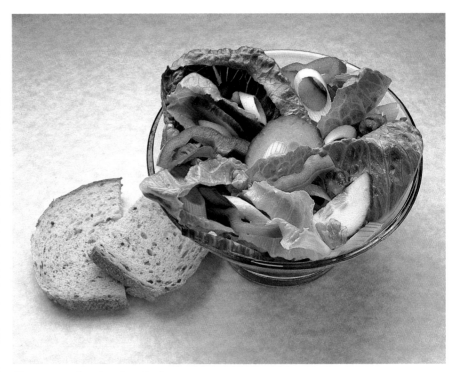

## Green and mixed salads

Be adventurous with your salads – limp old lettuce and tomato are too boring. Be generous, too: most saladstuff is so low in calories that you can eat as much as you fancy.

For your green salads, try exciting combinations of any of the following: chicory, celery, peppers, chopped cabbage, raw courgettes, raw flaked Brussels sprouts, chopped chives, parsley, watercress, lettuce, raw broccoli, raw cauliflower, raw French beans, spring onions, raw spinach, mustard and cress, sprouting seeds.

For your mixed salads, add any of the vegetables above to any of the following: tomatoes, grated carrot, radishes, raw mushrooms, fresh fruit.

## Savoury corn pie

Serves 5; 447 calories per serving

*4 oz/100 g polyunsaturated margarine*
*4 oz/100 g plain white flour*
*1-1½ tablespoons cold water*
*4 oz/100 g wholemeal flour*
*1 onion*
*12 oz/350 g can sweetcorn, drained*
*7 oz/200 g carton low fat Quark*
*2 eggs, beaten*
*dash skimmed milk*
*freshly ground black pepper*

Make pastry by putting margarine, white flour and water into a bowl. Stir in wholemeal flour and water into a bowl. Stir in wholemeal flour to form a dough. Knead on lightly floured surface, roll out, line a 7 in/18 cm flan tin and bake blind for 10-15 mins at Mark 6, 400 deg F, 200 deg C. Mix finely chopped onion with sweetcorn, Quark, eggs and skimmed milk. Season with pepper. Pour into pastry case and bake at Mark 6, 400 deg F, 200 deg C for 40-45 minutes.

## Spinach lasagne

Serves 4; 364 calories per serving

*2 onions, peeled and chopped*
*1 tablespoon polyunsaturated oil*
*2 lb/1 kg spinach, washed and trimmed*
*2 × 14 oz/400 g cans tomatoes*
*1 tablespoon tomato purée*
*pinch each dried oregano and basil*
*3 cloves garlic, peeled and chopped*
*freshly ground black pepper*
*6 oz/175 g cooked lasagne (green or white)*
*2 tablespoons grated Tendale cheddar*

Fry onions gently in oil until soft. Cook spinach over a low heat in a pan with a tight fitting lid, until tender. Place onion, spinach, tomatoes, tomato purée, herbs and garlic in blender for 1 minute. Return to pan and simmer for 15 minutes. Season. Place a thin layer of sauce in casserole. Top with layer of lasagne. Go on layering lasagne and sauce ending with layer of sauce. Sprinkle with cheese and cook, covered, at Mark 4, 350 deg F, 180 deg C for 40 minutes.

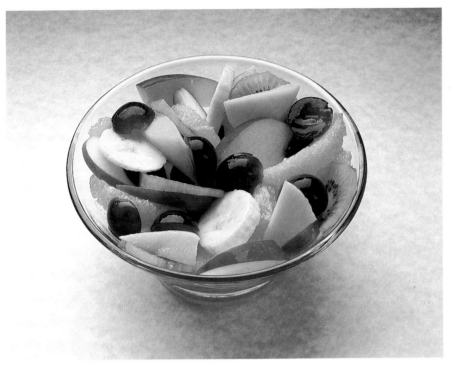

## Stuffed courgettes

Serves 1; 475 calories

*2 courgettes, topped and tailed*
*½ onion, peeled and finely chopped*
*½oz/15g polyunsaturated margarine*
*1oz/25g brown rice, cooked*
*1oz/25g soya beans, cooked*
*1 slice wholemeal bread, crumbed*
*1 teaspoon chopped parsley*
*freshly ground black pepper*
*1oz/25g Tendale cheddar, grated*

Cut courgettes in half horizontally and scoop out flesh. Blanch shells in boiling water for 1 min. Cool quickly. Fry onion in margarine, stir in rice, soya beans, breadcrumbs, parsley, seasoning and courgette flesh. Pile filling into each shell, top with grated cheese, cover with foil and bake at Mark 4, 350 deg F, 180 deg C for 20 minutes.

## Salmon loaf

Serves 1; 373 calories

*2oz/150g canned salmon, drained*
*2 slices wholemeal bread, crumbed*
*1 egg*
*2 teaspoons chopped onion*
*1 teaspoon chopped parsley*
*pinch tarragon*
*3 black olives, sliced*
*dash of lemon juice*

Combine all ingredients and put in ovenproof dish. Bake for 25 mins at Mark 6, 400 deg F, 200 deg. C for 20 minutes.

## Pizzas

See wholemeal bread recipe above for pizza base instructions. Halve recipe for 6 pizza bases. Top each base with 3 sliced tomatoes, then pile on any combination of the following: sliced mushrooms, green or red peppers, onion, mozzarella cheese, garlic, tuna, cooked lean bacon bits, olives, prawns. Freeze any you don't want to eat at once. Bake (fresh or frozen) at Mark 6, 400 deg F, 200 deg C for 30 minutes.

## Banana crunch slices

Makes 12; 176 calories per slice

*3oz/75g margarine or butter*
*3oz/75g dark soft brown or molasses sugar*
*2 small eggs*
*3oz/75g wholemeal flour*
*1½ teaspoons baking powder*
*2 small bananas, skinned and mashed*
*grated rind and juice of ½ lemon*
*2¼oz/65g walnut pieces, coarsely chopped*

Cream fat and sugar together until pale and fluffy. Slowly add beaten eggs, mixing 1 tablespoon flour in between each addition. Fold in remaining flour, baking powder, bananas and lemon rind and juice. Grease and line a 6-in/ 15-cm square tin and fill with mixture. Smooth top and sprinkle on nuts. Bake at Mark 5, 375 deg F, 190 deg C for about 20-25 mins. Cut into slices when still warm. Cool on wire tray.

## Fruit salad

Just chop up two or three different fruits (apple, banana and satsuma, for example). If you live with others, you can use more fruits without having to worry about left-overs going off. Melon, pineapple and oranges are good because they give you juice.

## Apple and walnut crumble

Makes 4; 352 calories per serving

*1lb/450g apples, peeled and cored*
*1oz/25g sugar*
*4oz/100g wholemeal flour*
*2oz/50g polyunsaturated margarine*
*¼ teaspoon ground ginger*
*1oz/25g walnuts, finely chopped*
*1oz/25g soft brown sugar*

Chop apples and cook gently with sugar until soft, in a saucepan with a tight-fitting lid. Place in an ovenproof dish and top with crumble mixture made by rubbing together flour and margarine and adding remaining ingredients. Bake at Mark 4, 350 deg F, 180 deg C for 40-50 mins.

## Bread and butter pudding

Serves 6; 175 calories per serving

*4 large thin slices wholemeal bread*
*knob polyunsaturated margarine*
*1oz/25g sultanas*
*4oz/100g peeled and grated apple*
*grated rind of 1 lemon*
*liquid sweetener to taste*
*1 pint/600ml skimmed milk*
*2 eggs*
*pinch ground nutmeg*

Spread bread thinly with margarine and cut into quarters. Arrange alternate layers of bread and fruit mixture in a 1½pt/1 litre ovenproof dish with a bread layer on bottom and top. Add a little sweetener to milk and beat in eggs. Pour over bread, making sure top slices are moistened. Lightly dust with nutmeg, place dish in a roasting tin half full of water and bake at Mark 5, 375 deg F, 190 deg C for about 40 mins or until golden.

# Firm-up and tone

To be totally effective in shaping you up, any diet has to combine with exercise. While all those pounds are dropping off, you need to firm up your muscles and whittle down your shape. You can speed up your metabolism; that is, lose weight faster and more effectively, by exercising 'aerobically'. Swimming, brisk walking, disco dancing, cycling and jogging are perfect. If you can't face any of these, try skipping in the back garden or running on the spot or up and down the stairs a couple of times. Half an hour three or four times a week should do.

But, if you haven't exercised recently, build up your sessions gradually, stopping for a rest when you are too puffed out to talk normally. Aerobic exercise is the only sort that, over time, will help to speed up your metabolism.

The exercises we have devised have a different purpose: they tone your body and help to shape it up. There's nothing to stop you doing both aerobic and firm-up exercises if you want to be really fit and shapely.

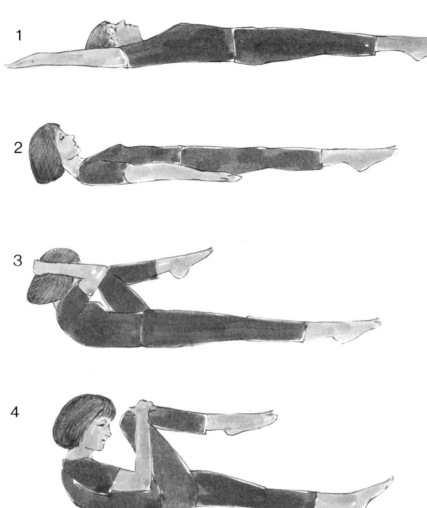

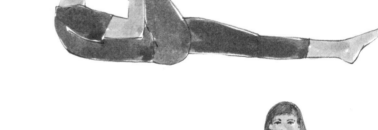

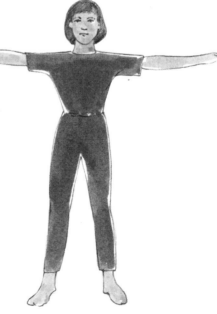

## Your firm-up routine

If you want to be really firm, try to fit in these exercises every day. If you find that you're stuck for time, concentrate on the ones for your particular weak-spot.

**1 THE STRETCH.** *Start your exercises with a thorough stretch from fingertips to toes, making sure your spine is straight and your body in line.*

**2 STOMACH.** *Lie on your back, hands by sides. Breathe out and raise head and shoulders to look at your toes. Breathe in as you slowly lower head to floor. Do five of these. As muscles strengthen, raise yourself higher until you are sitting upright. Always roll up your spine, never jerk up from hips.*

**3 WAIST.** *Keep same floor position and breathing as no.2. Hands behind head, raise right elbow and shoulder and left knee until they touch. Lower. Repeat four times and change sides. Repeat entire routine five times.*

**4 ABDOMEN.** *Start from same flat-on-floor position. Lift one leg – bent at the knee – and grasp is with both arms, raising head to touch knees. Hold and release. Repeat other side. Try 10 of these.*

**5 UPPER ARMS.** *Stand with feet a little apart and arms outstretched at shoulder level. Move entire arms in tiny circles. Do about 30 one way, then reverse direction, never letting arms drop from shoulder height. Try to do three minutes of this by pacing yourself to a fast reggae record.*

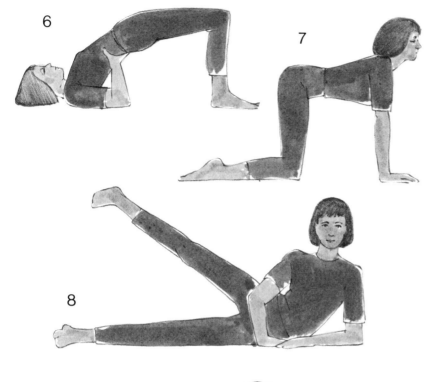

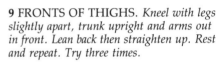

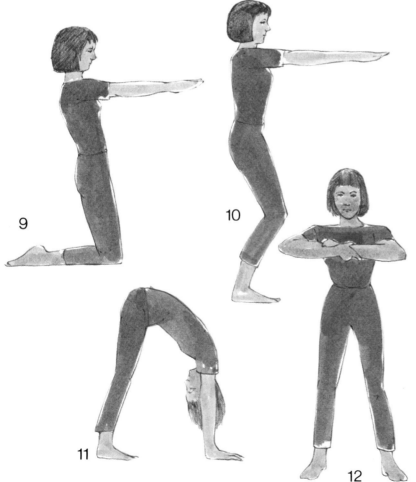

**6** BUTTOCKS. *Lie on floor with knees bent and feet apart. Now lift your pelvis, supporting back with your hands. Clench and relax one buttock 25 times, then the other, then both together. Relax, lower trunk and repeat, if you can, after a few moments.*

**7** BACK AND STOMACH. *Kneel on all fours, knees a little apart. Breathe in and push middle back and stomach towards the floor as you raise your head. Now breathe out, hump your back in the air and tuck your head down.*

**8** INNER LEGS. *Lie on one side, resting top part of body on one elbow. Lift upper leg, keeping it straight and turning toes towards floor. Lift and lower leg. Do about 12 each side.*

**9** FRONTS OF THIGHS. *Kneel with legs slightly apart, trunk upright and arms out in front. Lean back then straighten up. Rest and repeat. Try three times.*

**10** CALVES. *Stand with feet together, arms in front at shoulder level. Now bend knees, keeping trunk upright, and see how low you can get without heels rising from the floor. Hold, then return to standing position. Repeat five or more times.*

**11** BACKS OF THIGHS. *Bend forward from hips, moving straight legs close against a wall (support yourself with your hands on the floor or some telephone directories). Count to 10, then try to get your bottom closer to the wall.*

**12** BUST. *Bend elbows and grasp right forearm with left hand, left forearm with right hand. Hold them at shoulder height in front of you and push hard then relax, 30 times. Take a few seconds break and repeat.*

*Try to finish off each exercise session with five minutes or so of relaxation. Lie flat on the floor with feet a little apart and hands about 6 in/15 cm from your sides. Start at your toes and get every part of you to relax (even your mouth, tongue and eyes) so you seem to be sinking through the floor. And don't think about a thing! Come to life slowly by opening your eyes, turning on your right side and quietly coming to your feet.*

# Home gym

You don't have to go to the gym to tone up: however limited your space, you can exercise at home with easy-to-use fun equipment. The days when we all strove to look like underfed teenagers are happily long past. So if you are 10 stone of gently rounded, totally taut curves, don't suddenly seek a new shape.

Flab and the sudden additional half stone in the wrong places are the bits to beat. You can beat the bulges with our sensible eating plan (see page 60) and give your body a bit of home sport.

**On the rebound.** Jog and dance on a mini trampoline. It's great for the circulation and improving muscle tone on calves and thighs and strengthening ankles.

**Jump to it.** For an all-round pep up use a good skipping rope which doesn't tangle and can be adjusted to any length to suit your height. Apart from getting the circulation going, skipping tones and trims arms, buttocks and, in particular, legs.

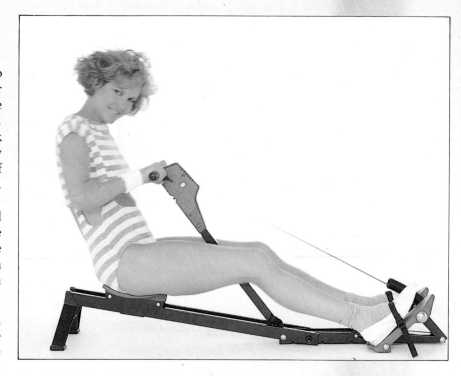

**Pulling power.** This 'Rower' exercises legs, arms, shoulders, back and stomach. One of the most physically demanding sports, rowing burns up the most calories so start your exercise plan *slowly* and follow the instructions and progress chart closely.

IMPORTANT. If you have any *back injury* or spinal weakness, consult your doctor or osteopath before tackling rowing. (The machine folds for storage.)

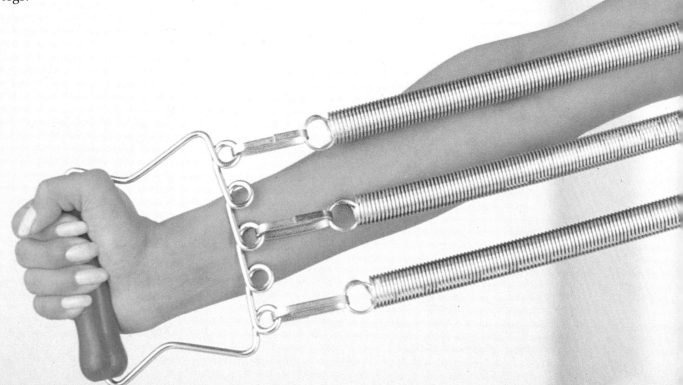

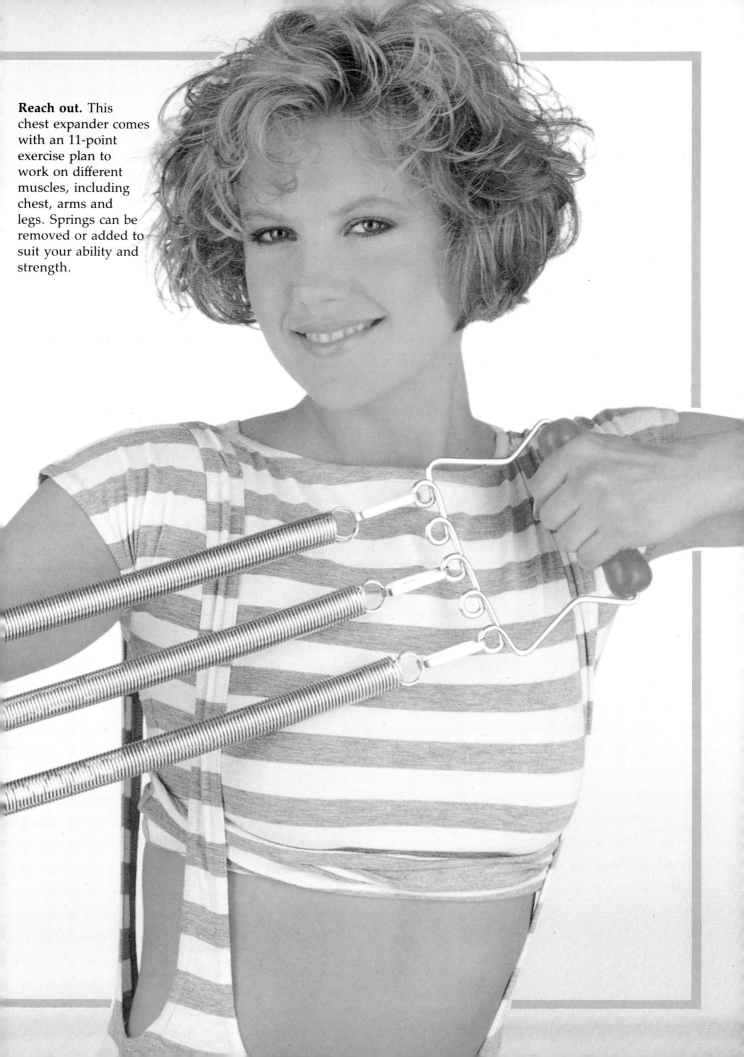

**Reach out.** This chest expander comes with an 11-point exercise plan to work on different muscles, including chest, arms and legs. Springs can be removed or added to suit your ability and strength.

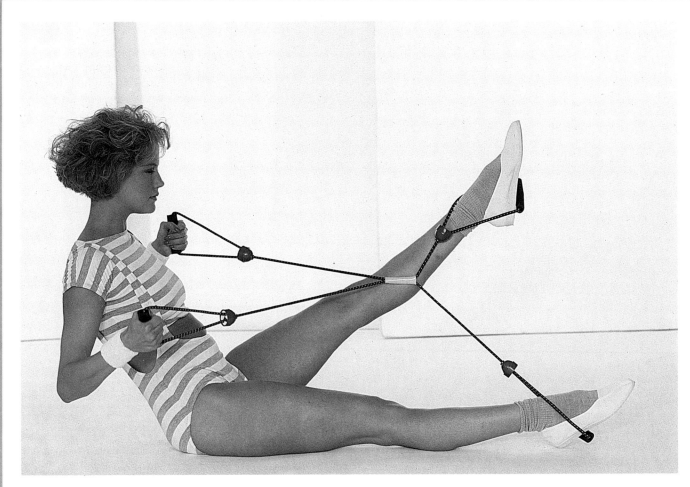

**Shape up.** You can stretch and strengthen practically every part of your body with a 'speedshaper'. Ideally, depending on which exercise plan you follow, you can concentrate on specific areas you want to tone up – bottoms, midriff, thighs and even upper arms.

**Chin up.** This chinning bar can be fixed in any doorway. It's great for strengthening arms, shoulders and improving posture.

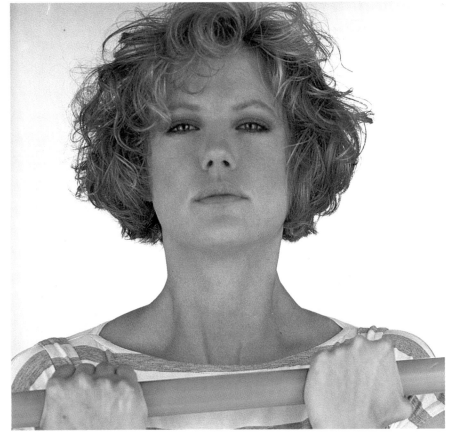

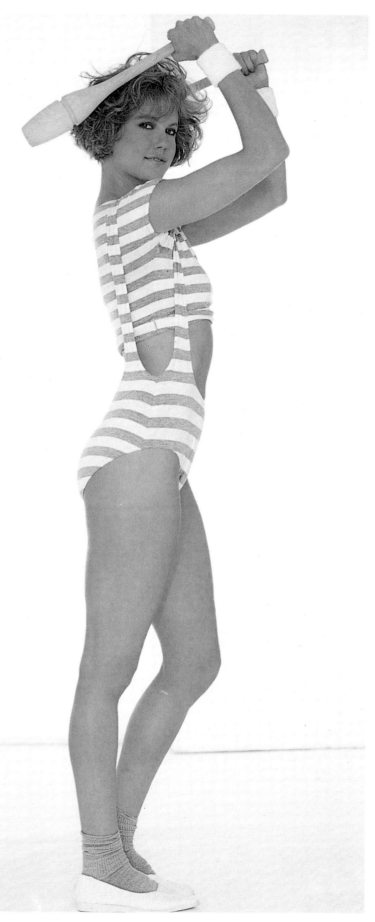

**In the swing.** Exercise clubs stretch and tone muscles from the waist up. Kits are available which include two beech clubs, cassette and exercise booklet.

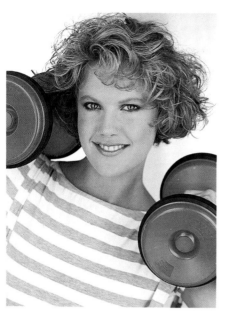

**Weighing in.** These dumb-bells are part of a complete work-out kit for rolling, lifting and stretching exercizes. (For more on weightlifting see page 76.)

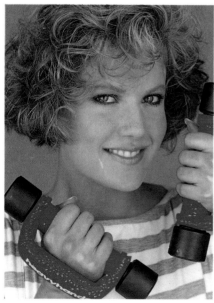

**Add weight.** Increase the value of your exercise routines by carrying handweights, while you run, walk and work out, to help you to burn up more energy.

# Weightlifting

At 35, do you look in the mirror and see droops and bulges where there shouldn't be any? This happened to Marilyn Luscombe, so she designed a series of moves and lifts to improve her figure. And as you can see, she succeeded – her body is now supple and firm.

When Marilyn was 35 she felt more like 60. She was constantly tired, depressed and on edge. After a demanding day at the office she would drag herself home and curl up, exhausted, with a dry Martini in front of the television.

## Transformation

Today, five years on, the difference is amazing. She has boundless energy; her skin is tanned and glowing; her eyes sparkle and she radiates confidence and good health. Sporty and high-fashion clothes have taken over from her former classic, understated wear. Dressed for her chosen sport – weightlifting – in a cut-away leotard, there's no surplus flesh at all on her body.

For Marilyn Luscombe, life really has begun at 40. And the magic route to her amazing transformation came about through **bodybuilding.** She has even written a book entitled *Designer Body* which explains what bodybuilding can do that aerobics and jogging can't: that is, it can actually change the shape of your body. 'I used to have really skinny, drooping shoulders,' said Marilyn, showing off her now broad, strong shoulders and the kind of figure you would normally only see on some fitter 19-year-old model.

Marilyn is well aware that bodybuilding conjures up images of unfeminine, flat-chested women with bulging biceps and over-developed thighs: There is a prejudice about bodybuilding for women – not least among women. Part of the trouble is that the public tend to see only examples of top women competitors in contest conditions. It's a very extreme look which can be quite shocking if you don't know anything about the sport.

'The average woman who weight-trains will never look like that . . . it takes years of really hard training and a specialized diet. There is a vast difference between bodybuilding as a competitive sport and as a hobby for toning and re-shaping the body. You will not develop huge muscles through bodybuilding unless you deliberately set out to do so. Anyway, very few women have the genetic potential to be a future Miss Olympia.

'I'm aiming my message at ordinary women who just want to improve their general fitness and appearance. It is not a miracle cure; it takes effort and commitment, but then there is no easy way to stay in shape. As you get older it gets harder because your metabolism slows down once you're over 30.'

Like many women she first turned to dieting. But she found that she was losing not only weight, but energy too, and her figure wasn't really improving. So she took up keep-fit classes. 'An awful lot of work for very small results. Then I met one of the gym instructors who had just arrived in England from California. She told me about bodybuilding – already very popular for women in the States, but few women in Britain had taken it up at that time.

## Food good

Undaunted, she joined Dave Prowse's gym. Within a few weeks she felt strong and loved the changes in her body. 'As I progressed, my shoulders became broader, my waist narrower, and my muscles toned up everywhere. it felt very, very good.'

So good, in fact, that she worked herself up to competition standard and was a finalist in two British Championships. And there were other benefits: 'It wasn't just my outward appearance that improved. I found that once I started exercising strenuously I was a hundred per cent healthier. My skin improved radically, so did my circulation – I used to be one of those people whose hands and feet were always freezing in the cold – but it's marvellous now. Because I have to be careful about my diet for bodybuilding, my digestion is much better. Everyone's system works so much more efficiently when one is fit and the more muscular you are the more calories you burn even while resting . . . and I find I sleep well and generally stay calmer.'

Marilyn speaks with an evangelical zeal. It's easy to forget that to achieve this feeling of well-being, she has to watch her diet and sweat it out for more than an hour four or five times a week in The Fitness Centre in London's Covent Garden. But there is no need, she says, to be quite such an enthusiast.

For those who want to give less time to the sport, it may help to know that you will see results after about six weeks of training for 20 minutes three times a week. It would take much longer than that to see results from aerobics or jogging.

'For the best results a balanced, low-fat diet is essential. One gram of fat produces nine calories, whereas one gram of carbohydrate or protein only produces four calories. Cutting your fat intake is the quickest way to reduce your body fat. Most women bodybuilders get their body fat levels down to around 14 per cent. The average woman carries at least 25 per cent. Bodybuilding is not some miracle cure-all, but you are able to control the level of improvement you achieve.'

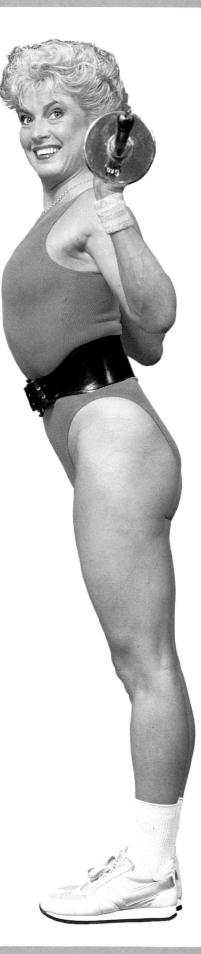

The upper part of women's bodies are generally weak (men have around 30 per cent more upper body muscle). Under upper arms are a high danger area.

The pull of gravity brings a natural droop to breasts over the years. Lifting weights strengthens pectorals – the chest muscles that support breasts.

The abdominal area is another naturally 'weak' spot. Lifting weights brings all-round tone, and helps to guard against flab.

Working on waist and buttocks also helps reduce heavy hip 'pads'.

Moves such as Good Mornings and Squats (see page 78) work on the glutals – the group of muscles which form the buttocks.

While the average woman does lots of running around and her lower legs are strengthened, thighs are often a problem area . . .lack of tone and lumpy fat deposits are no respecters of age. Banish flab with a combination of good nutrition, regular exercise and patience.

## Beginners' basics

Marilyn suggests that if you want to try out lifting weights, you can improvise with a couple of full food cans or empty washing-up liquid containers filled with sand or water, but you will soon progress beyond this stage. Most sports shops stock basic weight training equipment or you may find advertisements in magazines with mail order in local papers offering second-hand weights. If you start by training at home, you will need to buy a bar-bell with adjustable plates (the flat discs which range from $1\frac{1}{4}$ to 100 lb/570 g to 45 kg. They have a hole in the middle and can be fixed in different weight combinations on to the basic bar-bell) and a set of dumb-bells.

However, it is wise to seek expert tuition and supervision. The basic equipment to look for in a gym is a good range of bar-bells and dumb-bells – use fairly light ones if you are a beginner. There's no point in joining the type of gym where the dumb-bells start at 35 lb/16 kg because you will need some of the 3 to 5 lb/1·4 to 2·3 kg ones and bar-bells of 10, 15 and 20 lb/4·5, 6·8 and 9 kg. Make sure they rise in weight in easy stages, and that they don't stop at 50 lb/23 kg because you will get stronger very quickly and may soon be squatting 100 lb/45 kg or more!

IMPORTANT: *If you have any medical problem it is vital to get the all-clear from your doctor before weightlifting.*

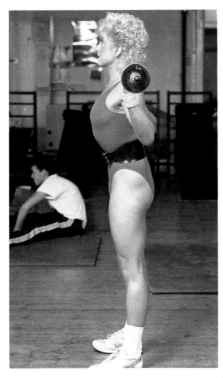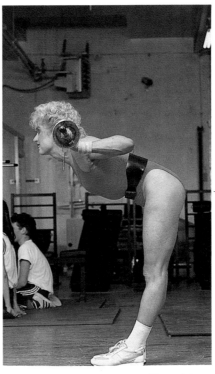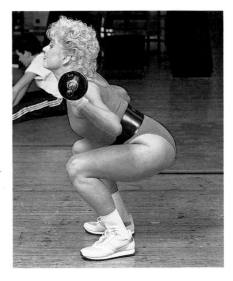

**Good Mornings.** *This exercise will strengthen lower back and firm buttocks. Stand with feet hip-width apart and a light bar-bell across your shoulders. Bend forward from hips, keeping back straight – not curved – until trunk is at right angles to legs. Get shoulders as low as you can and keep chin up throughout. Slowly return to the upright start position.*
**Please note:** *as this exercise is performed with straight legs, take extra care and use only light weights.*

**Squats.** *These are great for thighs. Place bar-bell across shoulders and grasp with hands equidistant between plates and shoulders. Keep feet flat on floor hip-width apart and toes slightly pointing outwards. Keep back flat and tense muscles. Looking at a point high in front of you, slowly bend at knees until thighs are parallel to the ground – see left. Never bend back by collapsing forwards. Return to standing position without lingering, exhaling as you do.*

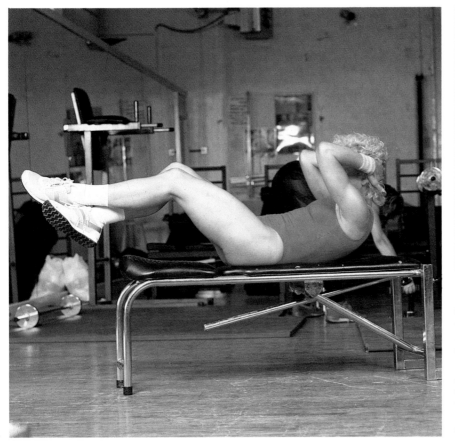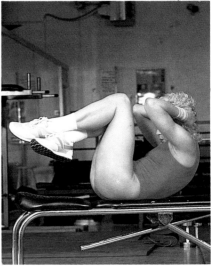

**Crunches.** *This exercise strengthens the abdomen. Do this on a heavy exercise bench or, failing this, the floor. Hold hands behind head and raise head and shoulders. Cross ankles slightly and bend knees (left) and lift them up towards head (above). Hold this position for the count of one. Lower legs slowly back down but don't lie back, collapse or relax. Keep tension in stomach. Repeat. Don't worry if you find this one very difficult in the early stages.*

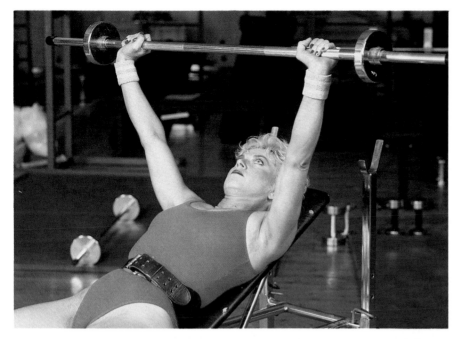

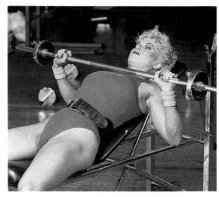

**Bench Press.** *For chest and arms, lie flat on a bench with feet on floor. Grasp bar-bell at shoulder width, lift and lock elbows (left). Lower bar slowly to chest (above), then push it up again powerfully – never arch back.*

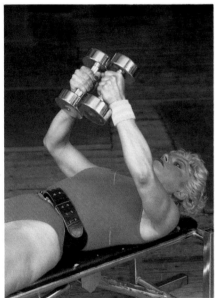

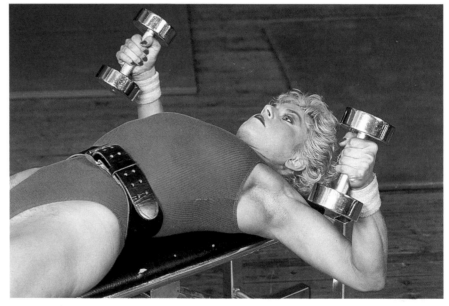

**Flat Flyes.** *For a firm bust, lie flat on bench with feet on floor. Extend arms with elbows bent and hold dumb-bells together above chest (see above). Move elbows and upper arms outwards (above right). Push weight back to starting position.*

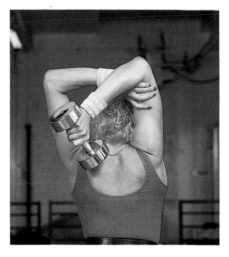

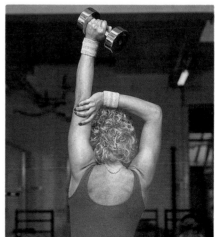

**For chest, shoulders, arms.** *Hold a light dumb-bell in hand with arm straight. Steady arm by grasping elbow (see right). Lower dumb-bell to opposite shoulder (far right). Pause. Push dumb-bell back to start position. Repeat other side.*

# Water works

Cleansing rituals with water have waxed and waned in popularity throughout the ages. The Romans went in at the deep end, turning bathing into a medicinal, social and sometimes a mixed affair. They turned the warm springs of Bath into a communal bath, and made Buxton a rest camp for their Legions.

The early Christian Church turned its back on bathing, and with the exception of a few monks – whose ice-cold dips were designed more for the benefit of the soul than the body – and the Crusaders – who imported the idea of steam baths – the British remained anti-water until the 19th century when the Regency and Victorian urge to purge helped to make bathing and 'taking the waters' fashionable. Britain's spa towns were popular with the rich and leisured, clamouring to be drenched, steamed and filled with 'curative' waters.

Spas are basically local waters with high mineral content believed to be beneficial in treating cases of illness, over-indulgence and neglect. The idea is that the waters are imbibed or their mineral content is absorbed through the skin during bathing.

While Continental spas like those using herbal remedies combined with hydrotherapy are thriving, Britain still puts its faith in chemical cures rather than water works. But British spa towns and villages have retained their charm and, with the current interest in natural remedies, water treatments are making a gentle comeback.

## Britain's Spa Towns
**Harrogate.** The Turkish baths are a marvellous example of Victorian 'Moorish' architecture. And, at The Royal Pump Room, you can buy water from the sulphur well.

**Bath.** This is Britain's oldest spa. The Pump Rooms attached to the old Roman Baths, offer spa water, music and food. The Pavilion in the grounds of The Royal Crescent Hotel has spa water pools and there are plans for developing an international spa with a range of hydrotherapy treatments.

**Royal Leamington Spa.** The local water, good for internal cleansing, is free at the Pump Room. Hydrotherapy/physiotherapy treatments are given in the therapeutic and vortex pool. However, these are available on medical recommendation only.

**Droitwich.** The 100 per-cent saturated salt water is great for people who need to ease their joints and limbs. The brine baths opened in 1985.

**Woodhall Spa.** This lovely, restful village was founded in the 19th century when the water was discovered to alleviate rheumatic conditions.

**Strathpeffer.** This unspoilt village in the Scottish Highlands has a natural sulphur well. The Pump Room reopened in 1985.

**Llandrindod Wells.** This small, pretty, mid-Wales town has a restored pump dispensing saline and magnesium water. If you suffer from anaemia, try the free chalybeate water.

**Cheltenham Spa.** The highly salty, mildly laxative waters of this elegant town are free at the Town Hall and the Pitville Pump Room.

**Malvern.** The famous water flows freely in the Hills and at St Anne's Well. The water is also available bottled.

**Royal Tunbridge Wells.** This charming town has a leisurely atmosphere and a 'dipper' at the well in the Pantiles to hand you – for a small sum – water rich in minerals, particularly iron.

**Buxton.** England's highest spa town is set in the Peak District National Park. Its attractive Pavilion complex boasts a modern spa water swimming pool. The water is also available bottled.

## Heat and water treatments
It's amazing what refreshing and body-stimulating beauty treatments you can find at your local Turkish baths if you can't afford the luxury of visiting a health farm or joining a health club.

**Steam baths.** The Turks and Russians used steam baths to cleanse and purify the body and mind. If you have one nearby, do try it. Steam and water are re-used in a succession of varying temperatures to induce perspiration which removes deep-down dirt and boosts the body's circulation.

Some baths offer a body shampoo massage which removes grime and dead surface skin as well as easing aches and pains and toning muscles.

A cool shower or cold plunge readjusts your skin and closes the pores. Always follow the suggested programme at your particular bath and don't stay in steam cabinets or hot rooms longer than is comfortable.

The sheer luxury of spending time on yourself is part of the pleasure of these baths. Allow at least two hours to get the full benefit from your visit.

**Saunas.** The Scandinavians, in particular the Finns, have long used saunas to keep the body 'spring cleaned' all year round. Instead of steam, saunas offer dry heat to stimulate the body to eliminate toxic wastes and energize the blood and lymph circulation. They help to make joints more supple while at the same time soothing muscles and refreshing the mind.

Most local health complexes offer saunas, and the market for home saunas is increasing.

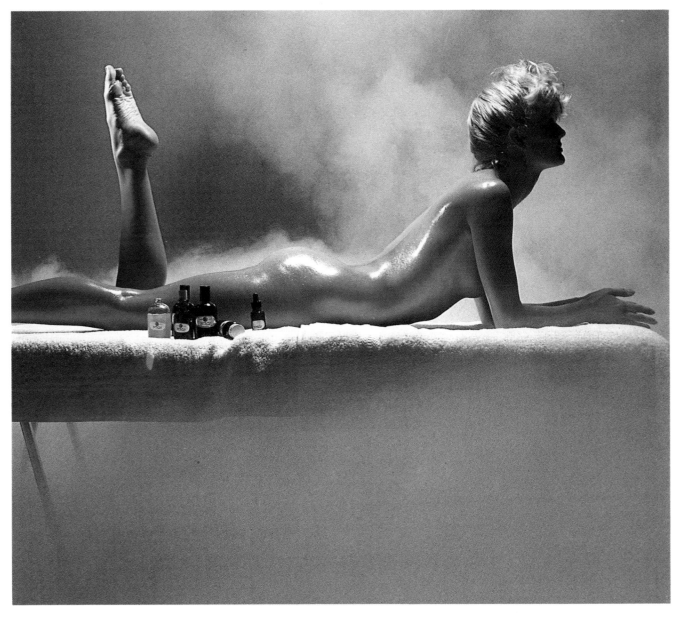

If you are not used to saunas, never rush at the heat in one long session – five to ten minutes at a time is enough to begin with, breaking to take short cold dips or showers in between. To start, always opt for the lower benches and lie down until you are used to the heat and can move to a higher bench. Never take a sauna after a meal or if you're on a liquid fast. Remove jewellery which can become too hot to handle and if you must wear something, make sure it is no more than a light towel. Rest for half an hour afterwards.

Saunas and steam baths are effective in getting rid of accumu-lated body wastes and in turn help to deter the build-up of cellulite (see page 86).

**Hydrotherapy.** Another external treatment for cellulite is hydro-therapy. The principles are those of massage by means of powerful jets of water directed onto the skin to improve circulation and gently break down the pockets of stub-born, trapped tissue. Apart from the overpowering jets, there are also hot and cold dips to stimulate the skin and circulation.

You could try adapting your own shower into a personal massage machine by fitting a shower head

*Give your body a once-a month treat with a sauna or a steam treatment – you'll be amazed at how clean you'll feel.*

with a wide range of settings, from regular spray to 9,000 pulsating jets of water a minute. Your existing system will probably need a booster pump.

Treatment tubs and Jacuzzis with swirling water relax the body and massage the muscles and joints. You just lie back and let the water pummel your body. They can be both invigorating and relaxing and most health farms and health clubs have one. (See our visit to a health farm, page 176.)

# Give your body a sporting chance

While you are trimming the fat and firming the flab, you will also get rid of all that mental and emotional tension if you take some exercise. And sport is a fun way to exercise. If you are game, choose an activity you enjoy – and if it includes fresh air and a little socializing with your friends, so much the better.

## Take a plunge

Swimming is the best all-over body toner and there are few sports so gentle and relaxing that you can do at your own pace and stroke. You'll burn as many as 600 calories an hour while firming legs, arms, breasts and working towards a flatter tummy. Swimmers have healthier lungs and heart so breathing is longer and deeper and oxygen intake is improved.

Swimming is classed as an aerobic sport (see page 70) which means that through deep breathing you will steadily improve the muscle tone in your upper body. Swimming is the perfect bust exercise beause the body is supported by the water. Another bonus is that it firms muscles but does *not* build them.

Swimming is suitable for anyone aged three months upwards. As the water takes the weight, disabled people are on equal terms with the able-bodied. The only time to hold back is if you have a cold, bronchitis or ear troubles. Wait until they have cleared up.

If you want to take up swimming as a sport, opt for an all-in one bathing suit rather than a bikini and you'll find you can duck and dive without losing those vital pieces.

## Pool exercises

**1** *Swing a leg to improve your hip hinging movement. Stand upright with one arm on pool edge. Swing right leg forward and back keeping left knee firm. Do 10 with each leg.*

**2** *Increase the flexibility of ankles by standing on one leg, stretching the other out in front of you. Rotate raised foot clockwise 10 times, then anticlockwise. Change legs.*

**3** *Improve posture and/or ease back problems by supporting your body with outstretched arms along pool side and pulling your stomach in as your spine straightens.*

**4** *Support yourself with arms on pool side. Stand on one leg. Make small circles with other leg gradually moving it out towards the side. Repeat the movement with other leg.*

**5** *Work on legs, waist and pelvis. Support your body with arms on pool side, keep your legs straight and move them in a circle. Do this 10 times, repeat in opposite direction.*

**6** *Supporting your weight on the pool side, bend your knees and bring them up towards your chest. Twist from the waist, moving bent legs first to the left, then to the right.*

**7** *Turn to face the pool side and rest your arms along the edge. Jump, moving your feet apart – about 3 ft/90 cm is enough – then together. Now speed it up – apart – together . . .*

**8** *Still facing the pool side, widen your feet to about 4 ft/1·2 m apart and lunge, first to one side then the other – with your knee bent.*

**9** *Stand sideways on to the pool side balancing yourself with one hand on edge. With feet a little apart raise opposite arm and bend towards pool edge. Repeat each side about 10 times.*

**10** *These exercises work well, but they're meant to be fun, so do a few regularly rather than a lot one day. This one is great for making the hips more supple, and the legs more flexible. Open legs as wide as possible, holding on to sides of pool with arms. Now scissor legs across in front of your body. Spread them again and repeat, varying the upper leg each time.*

**11** *Take a big beach ball and, using both hands, push it down in front of you 20 times, then repeat behind your back. Good for shoulders and chest.*

**12** *Stand with your legs a little apart so that you keep your balance. With straight arms press the ball down in the water and move it from one side to the other in semi-circles.*

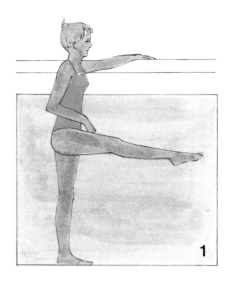

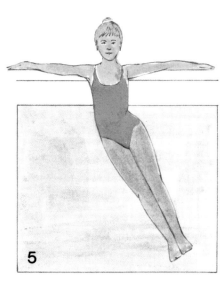

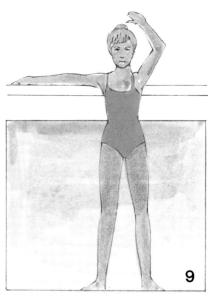

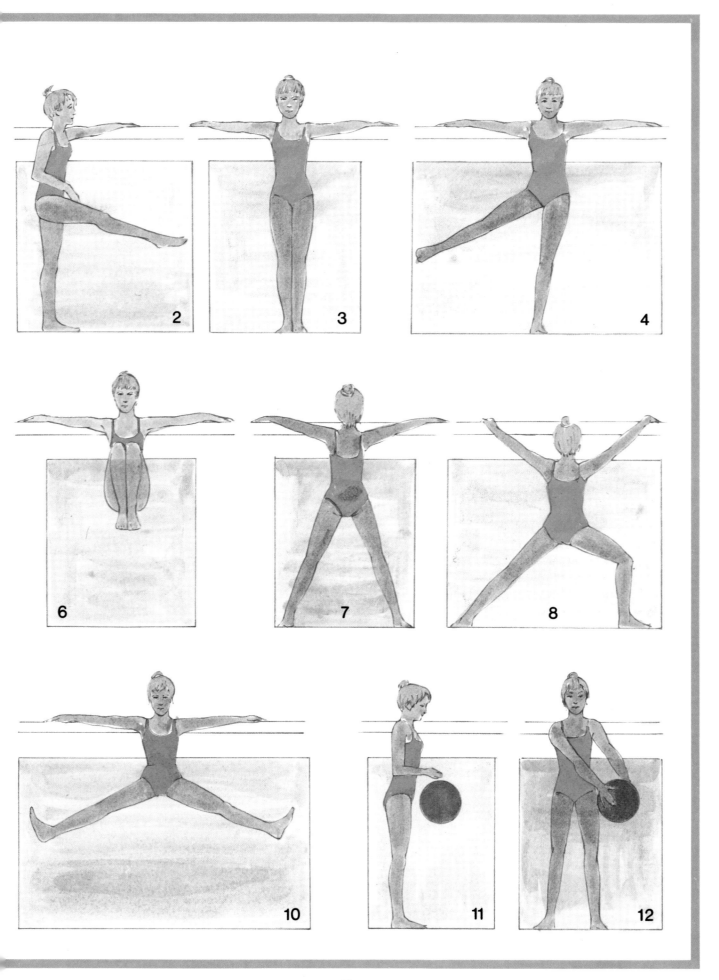

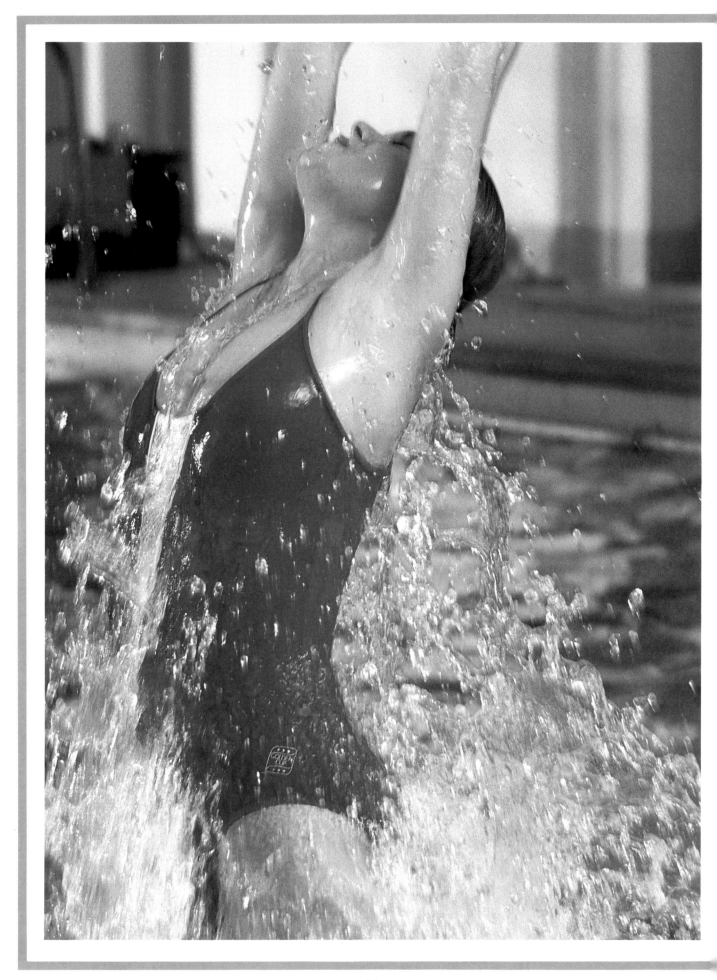

## Make it a fun run

New energy and vitality, a sexier body and better health are just three of the treats which lie in store for new joggers. The first step is the hardest. Like swimming, jogging can be one of those things you put off until tomorrow. But tomorrow never comes. This is why it's always a good idea to start with a friend or find out from your local authority, amateur athletics or recreational clubs if there is a jogging group in your area.

### Here are a few golden rules for joggers

● Don't wear men's running shoes. Women's running shoes are specially designed to deal with the narrower heel shape and instep of the female foot.

● Run in comfort. That means wearing loose, comfortable clothes, preferably made from a natural fibre – a cotton track suit bottom and T-shirt are perfect. Switch to cotton shorts when the weather warms up, and don't forget to wear cotton socks.

● Run in a sure, confident, but calm manner. Feet – heels first – should touch the ground firmly but lightly. Push each leg straight down to the ground. Don't kick your feet out to the side as you lift them off the ground. Take deep breaths, drawing oxygen right down into your lungs using your abdominal, not chest, muscles. Don't clench your fists. Swing your arms in a rhythm you find comfortable. Keep alert, particularly when running on grass where you may hit an uneven patch of ground.

*Exercising in water is a fun way to work out.*

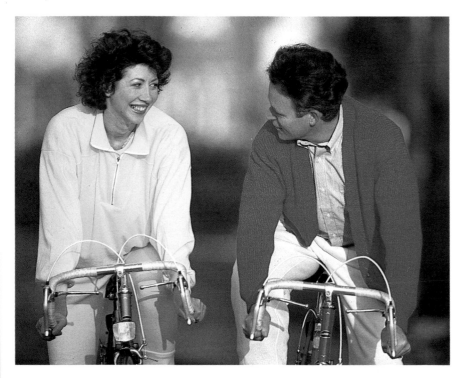

*Give the car a miss at weekends – biking's healthier!*

You may prefer to jog on your own or with your dog but there are three advantages to jogging with other people. The greatest is that it makes it easy to stick to a schedule – when you've arranged to meet someone in the street at 8 am, you can't lie in bed. The second advantage is that the friend helps to pace your jogging correctly. How? When you're learning to jog, you push your heart and lungs a bit to strengthen them, but you shouldn't do it too much or you'll put your health at risk. The easiest way to judge if you're at the right level of push is whether or not you are too breathless to talk. When talking gets too much, you're jogging too fast or too far. Slow down, walk a bit, or stop. The third advantage of jogging with somebody is that it's less embarrassing than jogging alone. New joggers feel that they may look peculiar or are doing it wrong. But if you're chatting, you'll forget about how you look.

Apart from giving you lots of fresh air and confidence, jogging leads to weight loss and body tone. It's great for trimming down bottom heavy women, firming up the thighs and trimming down the waist.

### On your bike

Cycling can help you to keep fit – and save on fares. The bicycle takes a lot of your body weight, so it's a suitable exercise even for the rather rounded, provided they're not going up huge hills. Cycling is relaxing (unless you're in city traffic), it builds up stamina and strength, helps to shape up your body (in particular legs), and is good for the heart, lungs and circulation.

### Serve up some aces

Tennis is a good excuse for running about in the fresh air. How much this game does for your heart, lungs, circulation and general strength and stamina will obviously depend on how well you play.

You'll develop strong muscle-tone in your legs and slim down your thighs as a spin-off bonus. Arms, too, will strengthen and upper arms lose flabbiness. You'll have stronger shoulders and an even stronger back. All this leads to better posture and lithe, confident walking. Tennis, like all sports, develops lungs and heart but, more than other sports, it demands concentration and sharp, swift reactions. Remember that the brain, like any other muscle, needs exercise.

Like other racket sports, it's great for the thighs, calves, hamstrings, hips, playing arm and shoulders and burns up approximately 500 calories per hour. The only disadvantage is that unless you are fairly fit beforehand, you could suffer serious strains on muscles and joints especially if you are volleying to win and over-exerting yourself.

Before tackling the game, try some pre-training like brisk walking or jogging to get your heart and leg muscles in shape. Then find a partner who is of a similar standard and, for a gentle introduction, try a set of doubles.

Get yourself some comfortable tennis togs and a good pair of tennis shoes that provide side-to-side flexibility for feet. Your local sports shop will advise on the type of racket to suit your play. Feel cool with cotton tennis knickers and wear a comfortable cotton sports bra which won't rub.

### Put your best foot forward

Walking may cost you no more than a matter of pennies for shoe leather. This can be a very genteel, peaceful pursuit, suitable for most bodies, or it can be strenuous if you stride out, join a club and head for the hills. Long regular walks will tone and trim muscles, build up endurance and work off a lot of tension.

### Take the reins

Horse-riding is still one of Britain's most popular pastimes but it can be expensive and difficult to pursue if you live in the middle of town. As a first-time rider you should not stay on a horse for more than half an hour since the strain on the back

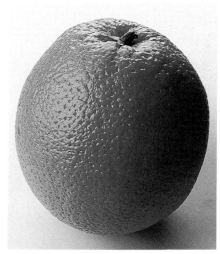

*'Peau d'orange' is the apt French description for cellulite! Keep it at bay with a healthy diet and plenty of exercise.*

and legs results in stiff joints and muscles. Even as a competent rider, you need lots of practice to keep in condition.

Horse-riding, as a sport, calls for a high level of endurance and courage. You're never considered a good rider until you've had a tumble or two! Riding strengthens neck, back, flattens tummy muscles, tones arms and builds muscles in legs.

You can ride in jeans, but you'll find it pretty uncomfortable as inside legs can be rubbed raw. It's far better to buy a pair of jodhpurs and wear an ordinary cotton shirt. A firm hat and high strong boots are essential.

### Tee-off

Golf is not solely for the rich. Municipal courses can make it great value for money. Golf can test your stamina – it's a long walk. It's great for co-ordination, flexibility and fresh air. It's a relaxing game for anyone aged 10 to 80, provided the wagers aren't too high or your temper threshold low! Private clubs, pro-training, your own set of golf clubs, however, can cost a lot of money.

IMPORTANT: If there's any doubt about your fitness, do take medical advice before indulging in any type of sport.

## Cellulite

If you suffer from 'cellulite' the (lumpy fat that accumulates on thighs and buttocks and, when pinched, dimples like orange peel), you're not alone. French statistics state that 80 per cent of women do. Caused by a build-up of toxic waste with cellular tissue, it is a condition linked with inefficient circulation, a rich diet, poor elimination of waste materials and too little exercise.

Cellulite is difficult to shift as fibrous, stringy buds secure it firmly in the fatty tissue but, if caught early enough, with the right diet and exercise it can be done. (If the condition is too far gone, cosmetic surgery is a possibility, see page 163.) Eat lots of celery and beetroot, drink apple and pear juice or liquidize lettuce leaves, celery sticks and parsley into a drink as all these eliminate toxic waste build-ups. Don't wear tight trousers as they restrict circulation.

Massaging areas of stubborn flesh is always beneficial. For thighs, work upwards from knee to groin, moving clenched knuckles in wide, circular sweeps. Repeat 20 times, twice a day. Use firm pinches over buttock and hip pads; finish by placing flats of palms at lower back and sweeping them round to stimulate kidney area. If you're a bit lazy on hand massage, then use a noduled rubber glove which takes all the work out of pummelling the stubborn area. Go gently when using gloves, or you'll end up black and blue. Most gloves come with total régimes of soaps, gels, and massage creams. Always use according to the instructions and combine your cellulite-bashing with a sensible eating plan and plenty of exercise.

### The cellulite-prone zone: bottoms and thighs

Whatever their size, bottoms slot into one of two categories. The apple shape curves out from the lower back, is firm and rounded and sweeps in at the top of the thigh with no droop. Apple shapes look good in the skimpiest of bikinis.

The pear shape is more typical of British women. The fat part of the buttocks is low and tends to droop where it meets the back thighs. Unfortunately, this shape wears badly with lack of exercise and a poor diet.

## Diet: the bottom line

It's no secret that eating properly is the key to good health. If you have to whittle away bulging buttocks, you need a low-fat, high-fibre diet (see pages 60 to 69), and you should drink lots of water to flush out those toxic wastes.

## Stride out and shape up

While buttocks and thighs may be overweight, they also have a lot of potential muscle beneath the fat to keep them firm. Jogging, walking, dancing, cycling, keep fit classes, in fact most forms of exercise will get the circulation going and, in turn, break down the deposits of fat (see pages 82 to 85).

## Beat saddle-bag hips

Here are some specific exercises you could try at home at least daily to trim you down.

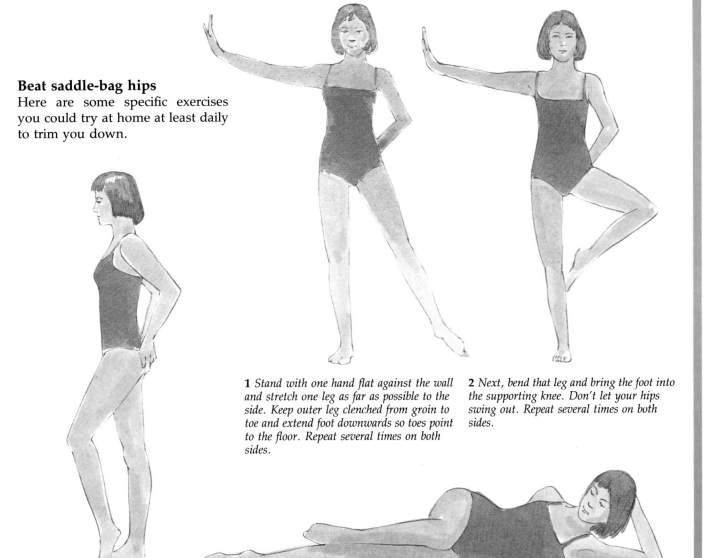

**1** *Stand with one hand flat against the wall and stretch one leg as far as possible to the side. Keep outer leg clenched from groin to toe and extend foot downwards so toes point to the floor. Repeat several times on both sides.*

**2** *Next, bend that leg and bring the foot into the supporting knee. Don't let your hips swing out. Repeat several times on both sides.*

**3** *Stand up straight with hands on buttocks and walk on the spot without lifting toes from the floor.*

**4** *Lie on one side with lower foot flat against the wall. Bring other foot up to your knee and stretch it down again. Repeat several times then roll over and do the same on the other side.*

*If you are having any form of medical treatment, check with your doctor before doing any extra sport or exercise.*

# Body Fresh

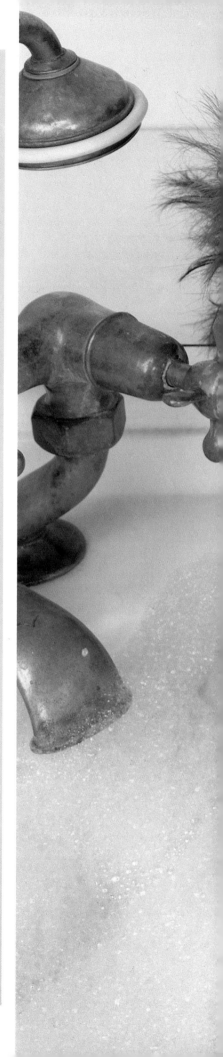

*There are lots of ways to stay clean and fresh: bathtime or showertime can be as relaxing or as invigorating as you like, depending on your mood. The days of good old-fashioned soap have gone. We're now seeing a wider than ever range of soaps to soothe or stimulate the skin – from those that can whisk off dry skin to glycerine-based soaps for moisturizing dry skins. And at the luxury end of the market you can lather up in a whole range of expensive fragrances.*

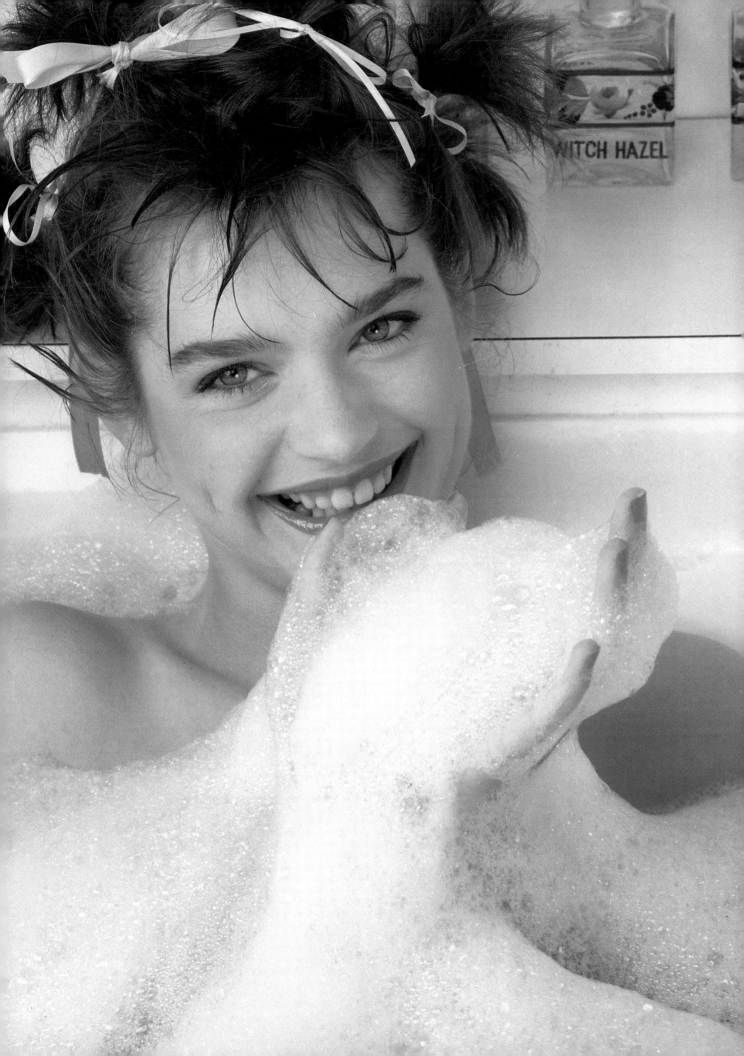

## Fresh new skin

You can now step out of the water with fresh new skin. Dermatologists call it exfoliation, which involves simply whisking off dead surface cells to reveal new skin. Now we can be smooth all over with all the numerous gadgets on the market from natural loofahs and body mitts to exfoliating creams which have gritty granules to polish the skin. You can even speed up skin's cell renewal using massage gloves or tone up cellulite-prone areas around the thighs by massaging to stimulate the circulation.

When it comes to staying fresh all day there's a product to suit everyone in the form of deodorants and anti-perspirants. Roll-ons are still popular although their formulas have been updated with more of a sporty image to suit the health and exercise boom which also sees the launch of unisex solid stick deodorants. Whichever one you opt for, you can guarantee that you'll find something to suit – even the more persistent sweat problems can be tackled successfully.

Perhaps one of your sexiest hidden assets is your perfume. Although it's invisible it can have a powerful effect on the senses and if you choose one to suit your own particular skin type, it will give you your own personal aromatic signature.

*After a warm bath, exfoliate your skin for a smooth, glowing look. Choose from the range of products on page 23.*

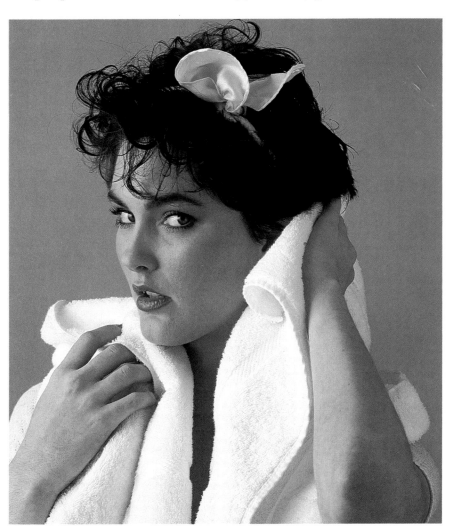

## Bathtime splash

Despite the increased use of quick-clean showers, there's still nothing like a soak in the bath for working on your mind and body – inside and out. Aromatic herbs, fragrances from the French Alps and oils from the East are just a few of the infusions you can add to the bath water.

*Never* soak in a hot, hot bath. At the very least it will sap your energy, encourage red, blotchy patches on your skin, increase or encourage any tendency to thread veins and the steam will do nothing for your hair. Hot water soaks can be dangerous if you are very overweight or have certain medical ailments.

Take a coolish bath to get you going in the morning or recharge your batteries if you are going out in the evening.

Increase the water temperature for a pre-bed, relaxing bath and wrap yourself in a soft, absorbent towel afterwards to pat yourself dry. You can turn on the taps for really hot water while adding your oils to get the best aroma but never plunge in straight away – leave the bath water until it is elbow hot but not too tepid.

### Setting the scene

Plan a relaxing bathroom colour scheme. Soothing colours are blues, pale pinks, greens and beiges, not brilliant whites or bright colours. Add a scattering of moisture-loving plants – ferns, for instance, lend a sanctuary air and add oxygen to the atmosphere. Soft lights, as opposed to spotlights, and sweet music also help. If you do not have a dimmer switch on any bright make-up lights, you could laze in the bath wearing an eyemask. Invest in a bath pillow that can be fixed in the most comfortable position to support your head and neck and, if you don't have a non-slip bath, use a

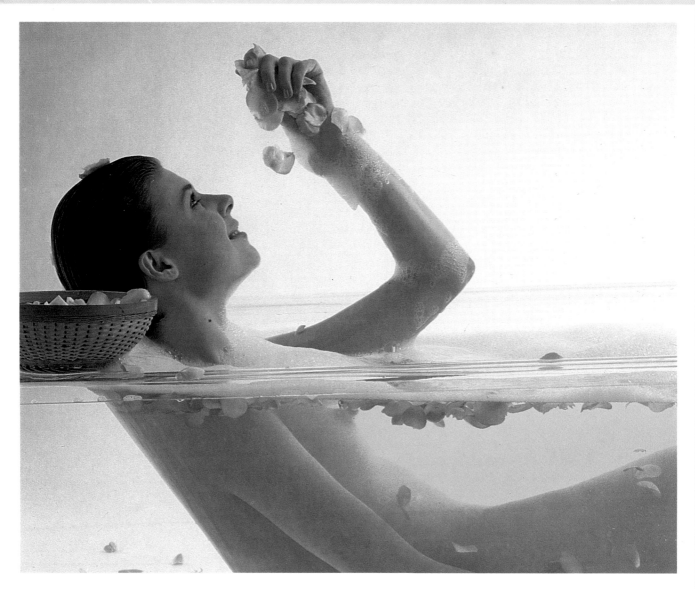

non-slip mat of fixed strips for safety and comfort. If you can't switch off your telephone bell, take it off the hook while you soak.

## Make your own bath additive

Delicate scents add to bathtime pleasure and many aromatic plants have a soothing effect on mind and body. A small selection of plants such as jasmine, lavender, bay, lemon balm, mint, rosemary, camomile, sage and calendula will give you the ingredients for a sweet-smelling, skin-smoothing bath. You can conjure up a wonderful fragrance and the prettiest picture if you just scatter the herbs in the water, but be careful not to clog up the drain. Avoid this by putting your herbs in a small drawstring bag that

you can hang under the hot water tap. You can re-use the bag by simply replacing the herbs and petals with fresh ones.

If you're feeling sluggish and/or your skin is rough and goose-pimply, put a little vegetable oil or almond oil and some coarse salt in the palm of your hand and rub it over your arms, legs, buttocks and stomach area before you get into the bath; the gritty salt will slough off dead surface skin cells and the oil will leave a moisturizing film all over your body.

Add a handful of Epsom Salts to your bath water if you're fighting off 'flu' migraine or the effects of too much wining and dining. Epsom Salts open the pores and help to eliminate toxins.

*Turn a bath into a sybaritic treat with herbs or oils.*

Add a wineglass of cider vinegar to the water to combat dry, flaky skin and help to restore the healthy, acid mantle.

## Commercial bath salts

Childhood memories of an over-powering smell from mother's or grandmother's bath salts can put many of us off using this useful, healthgiving and inexpensive additive to the water. But in line with the trend towards lighter perfumes and herbal ingredients, they now have a lighter fragrance, act as a water softener, and often contain body-beneficial mineral salts and plant extracts. For skincare, look out for those containing hops, horsechestnut, rosemary, or camomile. And some bath salts contain witchhazel, long recognized as a cooling and healing agent.

## The trouble with bubbles

While there's a staunch brigade that limits bath additives to a bar of soap, there's also an increasing number who come clean with a luxurious mass of bubbles.

Bubbles are also fun, particularly for younger children, but for older skins, remember that the foaming ingredients in bubble baths are based on detergents. If those images of washing-up liquid stripping grease from dirty dishes make you wonder what bubble baths do to your skin, remember that detergent is less violent than the caustic soda content of poor quality soaps. Most bubble baths now contain natural oils – almond, cocoa butter, palm, wheatgerm – to tip the balance on any drying tendencies, and there's an increasing move towards natural foamers with detergents based on products like coconut oil (rather than petroleum), so the detergent itself is not harsh.

## Milk baths

Failing a constant supply of asses *à la* Cleopatra for your milk dip, turn to one of the many bath products that soften water, cleanse the skin and are delicately fragrant, soothing and healing. Some milk baths on the market are made from vegetable and essential plant oils, others simply have a rich protein powder base designed to cleanse and condition.

## Bath oils

Some of the oil combinations to look for are: lavender, which is calming; rosemary, which is stimulating; citrus, which is freshening; and pine, which is refreshing after exercise.

Whichever method of coming clean you choose, make sure that your skin can stand the treatment.

If you have particularly dry skin, then some of the best body moisturizers on the market contain lovely fragrant essential oils that you can smooth on all over before getting into the bath.

# The big rub

If your skin is looking dull and grey, give it a polish with some of the scrubs and rubs now available, even the most stubborn skin on feet and elbows won't be hard to smooth off.

Skin tends to be sluggish in the cold winter months and you may not notice the tiny, flaking dead cells, particularly when your body is under cover. Skin renews itself by the minute but often needs a bit of help by means of exfoliation, which involves sloughing off the surface dead cells. Some dermatologists call it epidermabrasion and believe it's not always how you clean your face but when that is important.

Vigorous cleansing and massaging at night may feel relaxing and remove make-up, but the best time to slough off dead skin cells is first thing in the morning.

A useful gadget to take the chore out of exfoliation is a battery-operated facial brush. Its soft bristles and massagers clean deep down and stimulate the skin's circulation. Some kits include a pumice stone to smooth rough flaking skin.

A simpler and cheaper way of polishing facial skin is by means of a deep cleansing facial sponge, specially textured to lift off the hundreds of tiny cells. You simply use with soap and water and rinse your face well afterwards. Once these cells have been whisked away, new cells are encouraged to reach the surface.

## Face masks

These (see page 26) can tone, lift, cleanse, stimulate, moisturize and exfoliate. The deep-cleansing masks usually have a clay base which absorbs oils and lifts out dirt from the skin's pores. Also effective are the peel-off masks which dry like clear, rubbery plastic on skin and are normally applied with a brush. When dry, they are peeled off, taking the top layer of dead skin cells with them, and the face feels smooth and tightened.

Apart from the many masks on the market to whip off these dead skin cells, there are masses of different varieties of scrubs – for both face and body.

## Scrubs

A scrub improves the skin's texture by removing the top layer and stimulates the cells. Research has confirmed that new cells are born at exactly the same rate as old ones are lost, so you can aid your own skin-cell renewal process by massage and scrub.

The other advantage of polishing skin is that it makes it more receptive to any moisturizing or nourishing treatments afterwards – particularly if essential oils are used.

The creamy scrubs contain tiny grains or granules and are best applied to damp skin, allowed to settle and then rubbed off with a tissue. Some are water soluble so are easy to use in the shower. Oily and normal skins tend to benefit from a deep-cleansing scrub.

If you want to give your body a regular rub down, then opt for a loofah, friction mitt or massager to polish up larger areas of the body. All you need is your favourite soap and a bit of elbow grease. And don't forget elbows and feet – invest in a pumice stone (some are specially moulded), to tackle these stubborn skin areas.

To keep them fresh and clean, massagers and friction mitts should always be rinsed and hung up to dry.

Simple table salt, dampened in the palm of hand and rubbed over the skin in circular movements is

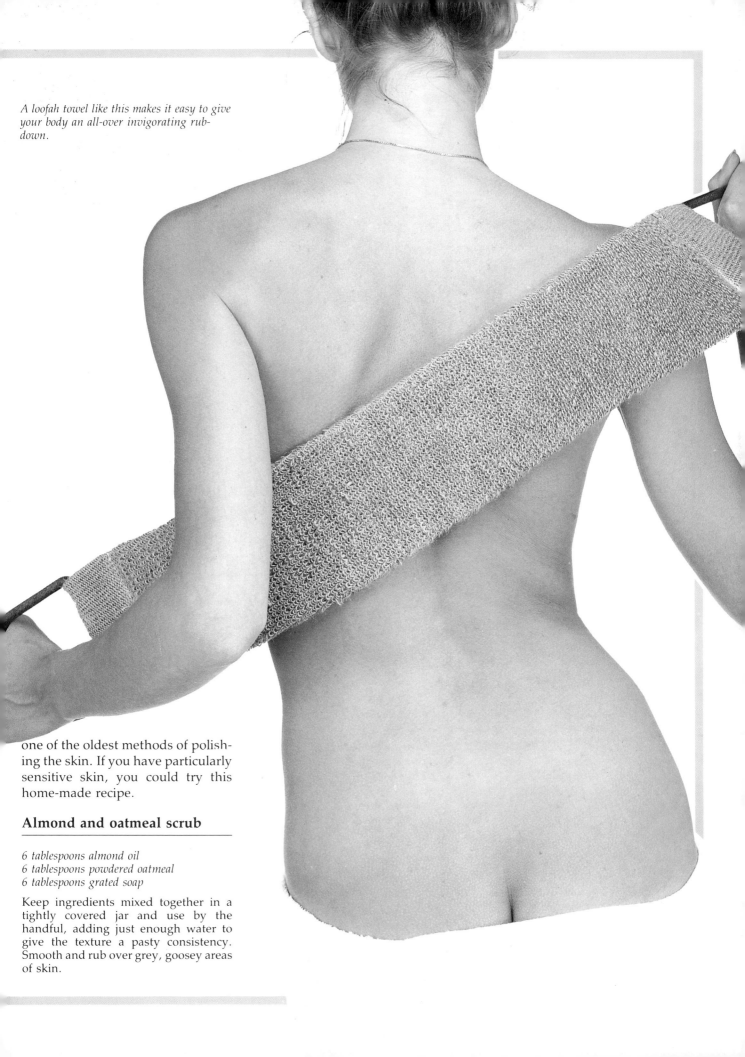

*A loofah towel like this makes it easy to give your body an all-over invigorating rub-down.*

one of the oldest methods of polishing the skin. If you have particularly sensitive skin, you could try this home-made recipe.

## Almond and oatmeal scrub

*6 tablespoons almond oil*
*6 tablespoons powdered oatmeal*
*6 tablespoons grated soap*

Keep ingredients mixed together in a tightly covered jar and use by the handful, adding just enough water to give the texture a pasty consistency. Smooth and rub over grey, goosey areas of skin.

# Lather up

Nice girls smell of nothing but good soap. Well that's what Grandma used to say, and with all the lovely soaps around, she could still be right.

## Soap as a cleanser

In recent years cleansing milks and lotions largely dismissed the old-fashioned soap and water routine as manufacturers and beauticians opted for the science of beauty which didn't include soap as a cleansing agent.

But old habits die hard and we've now done the full circle and are back into soaps. Today there's a soap to suit every skin type, a fragrance for every mood, at reasonable prices, and all kinds of stunning sculptured tablets to give your bathroom a touch of luxury.

Most soaps are alkaline, based on sodium hydroxide and fatty agents, and act as detergents – stripping the skin of dirt, oil and dead skin cells.

The only soaps that don't dry out the skin are those with a slightly acid pH balance (similar to that of the skin), or cleansing bars which are milder and less alkaline. But the use of soap and water is still a controversial issue with dermatologists.

The oily and fatty elements in the superficial skin cells help to retain moisture, and some believe that soap breaks these down, making the skin dry, sore and flaky. But Dr Vernon Coleman, dermatologist, declares: 'Soap and water are the best products for cleansing the skin.' And Erno Laszlo, one of the top skin preparation manufacturers, says: 'A skin washed with cream can never be clean.'

Despite differences in opinion, seven out of ten women still use a soap. All soaps form a scum, whatever they are, and whatever the price. So the skin must be well rinsed after using soap, or the pores will become clogged. The water

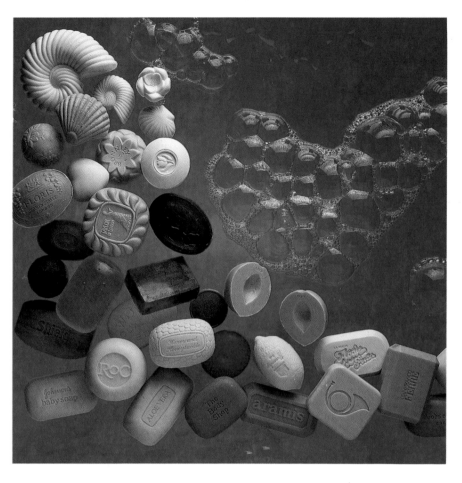

determines the amount of scum that forms. In hard water, soap forms a scum of insoluble calcium salts, but soft water doesn't contain calcium, which is why it forms very little scum.

## Which product?

Soaps with added moisturizing ingredients are good for drier skins – particularly those that contain jojoba. The oil from the jojoba nut is a natural lubricant and is recommended for children and those with sensitive skin.

The herbal extract taken from the succulent tropical plant *Aloe vera* is also a natural moisturizer and emollient and is ideal for dry skins.

Pears' transparent soap contains no harsh additives and has been made from natural oils and pure glycerine for nearly 200 years.

If your skin tends to be on the oily side, look out for soaps with specific formulations to control grease. Spot-free greasy skins benefit from

*Use glass jars full of soaps as a decorative accessory to your bathroom.*

the slightly abrasive action of oatmeal grained soaps that whisk off the superficial dead skin cells and stimulate the skin.

For those who prefer not to use soap on the face, it's worth trying cleansing bars. Vichy's Aqua-Tendra dermatological cleansing bar is guaranteed soap-free, perfect for delicate, sensitive skins.

RoC's Compact Facial Cleanser is neither a soap nor a cleansing bar, but a solidified cleansing milk to use with water. It's hypo-allergenic and perfume-free.

Whichever method of cleansing you choose, be sure to use it twice daily. And no matter which product you get into a lather over, remember it's only the first step to healthy skin. Diet (plenty of fresh fruit and vegetables), fresh air and regular exercise all contribute to that healthy glow.

# Keep your cool

Staying fresh isn't just a personal issue any more – it's big business. Of all the deodorants and anti-perspirants on the market, aerosols are the favourites (with the men too) closely followed by roll-ons. But whether you prefer the good old-fashioned roll-on or the new solid sticks, here's how you can stay cool when the heat's on.

We all sweat – it's a normal healthy function – but there are certain circumstances in which we sweat more than we should, thus making it socially unacceptable. Apart from the additional stresses of modern living, we're wearing more man-made fibres which, un-like linens and cottons, don't allow our bodies to breath efficiently, so perspiration is trapped and odour results.

## What is sweat?
There are two kinds of sweat. One is undetectable; the other needs deodorising.

The undetectable type of sweat is secreted from the eccrine sweat glands, found mainly on palms of hands and soles of feet, the face and underarms. The perspiration these glands secrete is 99·5 per cent salt and water.

The apocrine glands, mainly under the arms and in the genital areas, are formed from hair follicles. They are much larger than eccrine glands and the secretion is heavier. These glands represent secondary sex characteristics and are more numerous in women than men. The perspiration from these glands, in addition to salt and water, contains fatty matter and, when trapped in enclosed areas, soon develops an unpleasant odour caused by bac-terial action.

## When do we perspire?
Eccrine glands mainly regulate body heat but they also respond to stimuli of fear, shame, anger or embarrassment. Mental stress, hot spicy foods, alcohol and heat trigger them off. The apocrine glands do not respond to heat. They are formed during puberty and are linked with hormone changes. They do, however, respond to fear, emotional stress, upset and tension, and are more active during men-struation.

An anti-perspirant is designed to prevent or suppress an excess of sweat from both eccrine and apocrine glands for varying lengths of time, according to the formula. And, if there is any minor level of sec-retions, this is diffused by the astringent aluminium salts found in many products.

Deodorants do *not* suppress the flow of sweat. They simply stop the development of odour with power-ful bacteriocides which cling to the skin's surface. An antiperspirant/deodorant combines protection against wetness and odour.

It has been argued that stopping the body from sweating is un-healthy. This is not true, since if you're only stopping a certain amount of offensive sweat from a small area under the arms, it can hardly cause a total blockage.

## Which product?
There are specific formulas in the shape of aerosol sprays, roll-ons, creams and sticks which can meet most requirements, including spec-ific creams to deal with excessive perspiration problems. Some prod-ucts are fragrance-free. Some anti-perspirants may work on one per-son but not on another.

Those with sensitive skins that become inflamed easily should try the ranges which are free of harsh bacteriocides.

## Sweat check
If you perspire very heavily, then it's worth trying a product from a range which specializes in this problem. Such ranges include roll-ons, perfumed, and an unperfumed cream. The makers claim that the formula encourages the sweat ducts to direct their fluid secretions into the deeper layers of the skin where the other body processes get to work to eliminate them. Active agents go to work within the sweat ducts making them re-absorb the perspiration as it is produced. It doesn't permanently block the nat-ural flow, only controls it.

Look out for ranges with strong double-action formulae with an anti-perspirant and a deodorant combined. They work by slowing down the eccrine and apocrine sweating process.

---

### Strong attitudes to BO
A survey conducted by Gallup in 1985, from more than a thousand interviews across Britain, showed that people's attitudes to personal body odour could strongly affect their love-life.

The survey showed that 53 per cent of people worry about working with a 'pongy' person and 58 per cent said they would think twice about going into a shop where an assistant had 'BO'.

Nearly a quarter of those interviewed said BO could put them off a prospective girlfriend or boyfriend. Nearer to home, 12 per cent revealed that they had a friend or relative whom they considered had an odour problem. Of these 32 per cent had consciously avoided the person, while nearly half had at some time felt it necessary to talk to them about their problem. On public transport, 55 per cent of people interviewed said that they had at some time moved away from another passenger because they smelt so much.

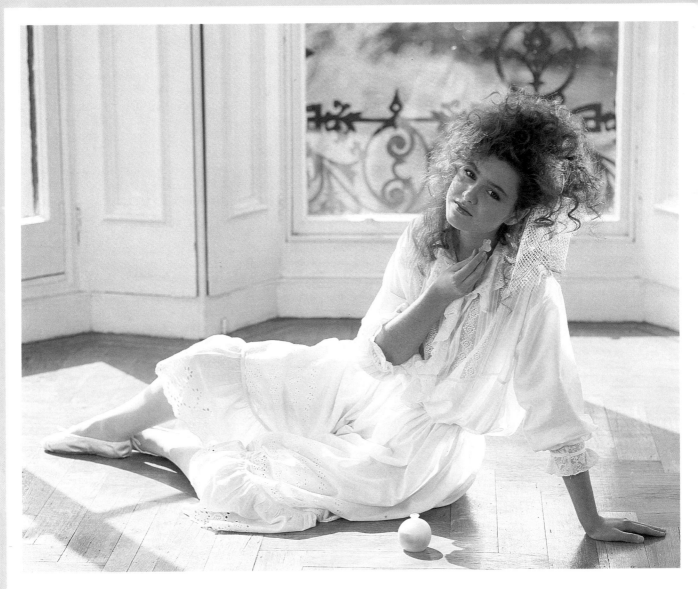

# The power of perfume

You can't see it or taste it, but scent can have a powerful effect on the senses if it's worn in the right places – and wearing it is an art. There's a special fragrance to suit your own body chemistry; here's how to identify it.

## Your fragrance

Consider for a moment the perfumier who so lovingly blends flowers, oils, roots, grasses and fixatives to make what will become a distinctive aromatic signature. He or she will tell you that no single fragrance can smell the same on any two women and that a woman's chemistry is the magic ingredient which will dictate how others pick up her scent. That's why, when you choose a perfume you should never choose it because it smells good on a friend or in the bottle. What you must do is whiff, sniff and experiment with a whole range of fragrances until you get wind of one or two that are, in your judgement, decidedly you.

When you buy, forget about buying in bulk to save money because as soon as the bottle of scent is opened and exposed to the air, the ageing process begins. This is why you should always store it in a cool, dark place and replace the top tightly after use.

Fragrances fall into five categories: Floral, Oriental, Green, Citrus, or Modern.

*Use fragrance every day – not just for special occasions.*

**The Florals** based on blossoms, were the pioneer fragrances. In the 19th century, women crushed rose petals, lavender, violets, hyacinths and lily-of-the-valley to make their own toilet waters. Today, florals are usually a harmonious light blend of many flowers. Florals are most suitable for young girls, grandmothers and great-aunts who love the sweet smelling, old-fashioned flowers of cottage gardens.

**The Orientals** are full-bodied and sultry. Here their bases are drawn from musk, ambergris, patchouli and civet. They are considered rich, heavy and sensual.

**The Greens** are woody, mossy and based on fern, sandalwood, rosewood and oakmoss. They are best worn by women who find the oriental fragrances too heady for them but who like a warm, refined smell with a note of the invigorating outdoors.

**The Citruses,** which became the cult of the late Seventies, take their base from tangy lemon and orange blossom. They are young at heart, fresh, clear and sharp. They are for the women who love the outdoors, sports, and who want always to feel fresh and crisp.

**The Moderns** can be a mix of citrus, floral or fruit    They are epitomized by Revlon's Charlie which made a big hit in the early Seventies. Many of the modern fragrances are synthetically-made replicas of traditional ingredients blended with new aromatic notes.

## Choosing your scent

Start at a cosmetic counter and learn to develop a nose. You don't need long – five minutes will do – but remember your nose becomes 'confused' after trying the third fragrance, so don't be too ambitious. Choose one, spray it on your wrists, rub them together, wave them in the air. Sniff. Do you like it? Wait a little longer and sniff again.

Every perfume has a range of three 'notes'. The first note, the top note, is the one you pick up the moment the perfume touches the skin. After about 10 minutes when the fragrance has warmed and mixed with the chemistry in your skin, you will receive the 'middle notes'. It is now that one fragrance will begin to smell totally different on two women.

When these middle notes fade after an hour or two, the rich 'base notes' come to the fore. If you don't like these base notes, you should try another fragrance.

## How strong?

Scent can come in many forms: as a concentrate, eau de toilette (also called toilet water), and in solid form (creams and sticks).

The concentrate is the expensive, top of the market choice and is dabbed on the warm pulse points of the skin – behind the ears, on the wrists. If you prefer to splash or spray your fragrance then eau de toilette is best for you. Solid perfume is made by suspending the fragrance in beeswax and body lotions. It can be applied to backs of wrists and insides of elbows and is ideal for the summer as it has a pleasant cooling effect.

Your fragrance is too strong if you are still overpowered by it after 10 minutes. Whether you choose a concentrate or eau de toilette, you should not expect your scent to last more than four hours.

Remember that you will hamper the impact if you smoke, because the nicotine absorbed in your body affects the body chemistry and therefore the oils in your skin. Equally, medications can change the way a fragrance reacts on your skin, especially anti-depressants which can decrease the body's natural perspiration. So, if suddenly your favourite perfume no longer seems to work for you consider any changes that your body has undergone. Scent is your personal message.

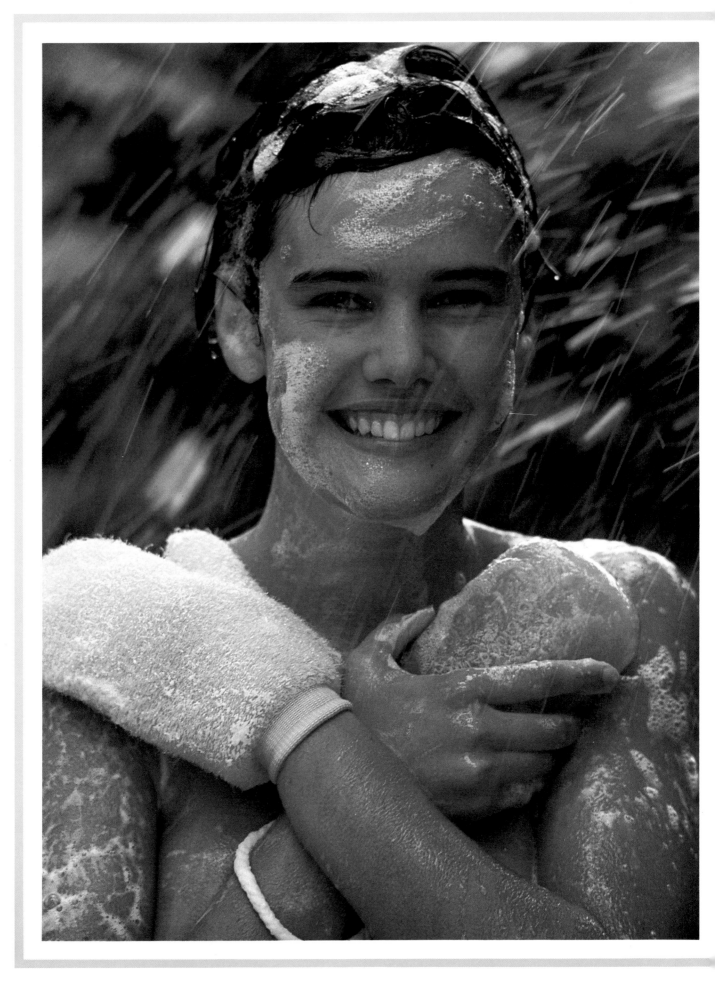

# Ten point plan for freshness

**1** Have a bath, shower or all-over wash each day. Your place of work can make you hot and sticky, especially in the summer, so keep a toilet bag handy with moist freshen-up tissues, deodorant and/or anti-perspirant for extra back-up during the day.

**2** Don't give sweat a chance to linger – keep underarms free of hair (see page 147). A light dusting of talc also helps.

**3** Deodorants and/or anti-perspirants are a must for underarms. Find one that suits you – effectiveness of a product varies from person to person.

**4** Wear fresh clothes, especially undies, every day. Choose natural fibres like cotton and linen when-ever possible. Unlike man-made fibres, they absorb any dampness and are not nearly so likely to become smelly. Nylon tights make you sweat, so avoid them when you can, particularly in the summer. Stockings are healthier, too – try hold-ups if you don't like wearing a suspender belt.

**5** If you have an underarm wet-patch problem, loose-fitting sleeves should do the trick. In fact, avoid anything too tight around under-arms, waist, legs or crotch.

**6** Steer clear of spicy food such as curries – they raise the temperature and create temporary sweating. Similarly, both alcohol and smoking speed up the metabolic rate which, in turn, activates the sweat glands.

**7** Nervous tension triggers off those glands, too. For some people sweaty hands, for instance, can be a night-

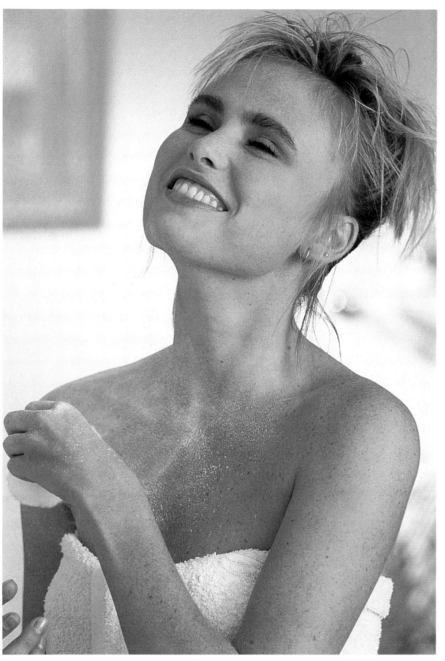

*Lather up your favourite soap and friction mitt to polish your skin, then finish off summer baths or showers with a cold water splash.*

mare. Staying stress-free is easier said than done but some people swear by yoga techniques. If you have time, relax for 10 minutes with your feet up. Breathe deeply and evenly and clear all the problems from your mind. The more you practise a serene state of mind, the healthier you become. And the fresher you stay.

**8** Learn some keep-cool tricks. All-over body sprays are a good start. Mineral water sprays for face and wrists bring instant relief. Running your hands and feet under cold

*Echo your favourite fragrance by using matching talc and soap.*

water is blissful, too. And keep your hair off face and neck.

**9** Being fresh and sweet-smelling go hand in hand. Using matching soap, talc and cologne creates an aura of freshness.

**10** Don't let a worrying problem continue. Ask your doctor for re-assurance and advice; worrying in itself can make you hot and both-ered anyway.

# Hair Care

*There isn't a woman in the world who is totally happy with her hair all the time. Your hair can reflect not only your state of health but also your moods. You only have to suffer from a 'flu virus or a cold and your hair loses its bounce and collapses in a matter of hours.*

*Knowing your hair's strengths and limitations is the first step towards keeping it in peak condition – it's almost like knowing how much food you can eat before you put on weight. There's no point in trying to grow hair long, for instance, when it can't take the strain.*

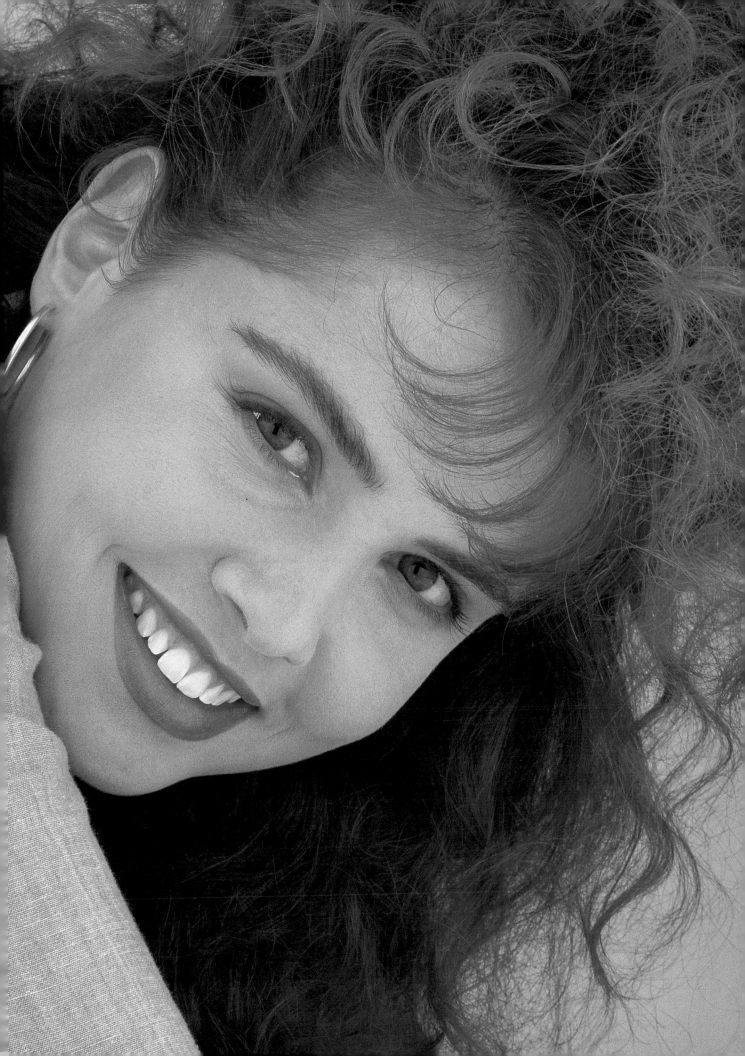

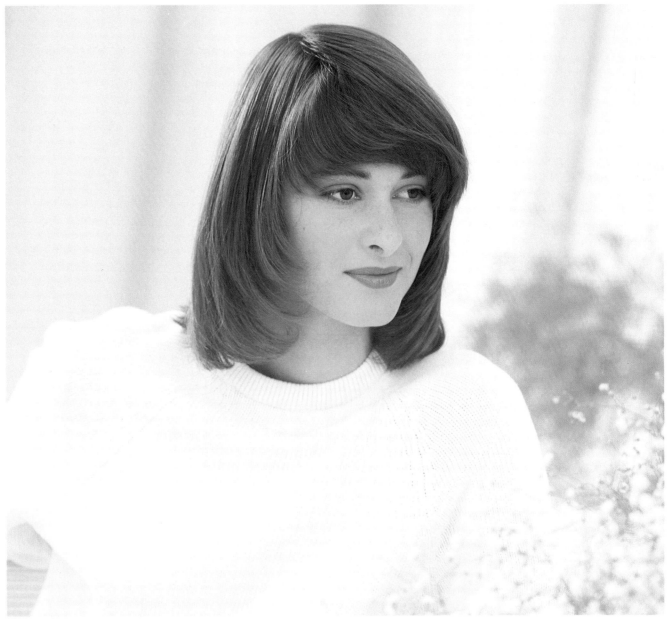

## Cutting

A good haircut not only boosts your confidence but enhances your hair's shape, style and condition. Cutting hair won't make it grow any faster; it simply makes it look bouncier and healthier. Snipping off the thin split ends makes the remainder look thicker.

Hair should be cut every six to eight weeks, although with some hair types a style can last longer, depending on the rate of growth. Once the hair has been styled into a well-cut shape, it will need no more than a regular trim.

How do you find a good hairdresser? A good hairdresser is someone who actually styles your hair to suit your face and lifestyle. Have a discussion with your hairdresser. Tell him or her about your job and your hobbies, and how much time you have to spend on your hair. It helps to take along magazine cuttings of styles you like and the shape you want.

However, do take your hairdresser's advice on whether your face is best suited to a short cut or if you need to let that bob reach chin length. Have confidence, not only in yourself, but in your stylist too.

*Whatever your budget a cut or good trim is essential every six weeks or so for good looking hair.*

## Know your hair type

Hair varies considerably from person to person in colour, type, texture, and shape.

**Colour** is determined genetically and once baby hair has gone, the hereditary colour shows through.

**Type** is determined by whether your hair is dry, oily, normal or combination, and whether it is straight, wavy or curly.

**Texture** is determined by whether you have fine flyaway, normal, or thick/coarse hair.

**Shape** is determined by how your hair naturally grows – the position of the hairline and whether the hair falls away from or over the face. The crown at the top of the head determines whether hair grows backwards or forwards.

### The different hair types:

**Dry hair** is usually coarse and becomes drier with age. Scalp oil treatments using almond or jojoba oil applied before shampooing will help.

**Greasy hair** can vary according to life cycles, such as hormonal imbalances, particularly during adolescence, and environmental conditions like the weather and central heating. It tends to look dull, lank and won't hold a style.

Greasy hair will benefit from frequent shampooing and a light body perm to dry out the oil.

**Normal hair** is healthy, glossy, can be fine or flyaway but always has a natural bounce and sheen.

**Combination hair** has dry ends and greasy roots – usually caused by rough handling. Have hair trimmed frequently and condition the ends.

*The secret of a good shampoo is in the rinsing – you can never rinse enough.*

# Shampooing

The belief that washing hair every day dries out the hair and scalp no longer holds true – not with today's technology. The gentle formula shampoos remove only dirt and grime and don't affect the scalp's natural secretion of oils.

You can shampoo your hair every day – whatever your hair type. But remember that shampoo only cleans hair; it won't repair or alter overactive oil glands. The average person shampoos every two to

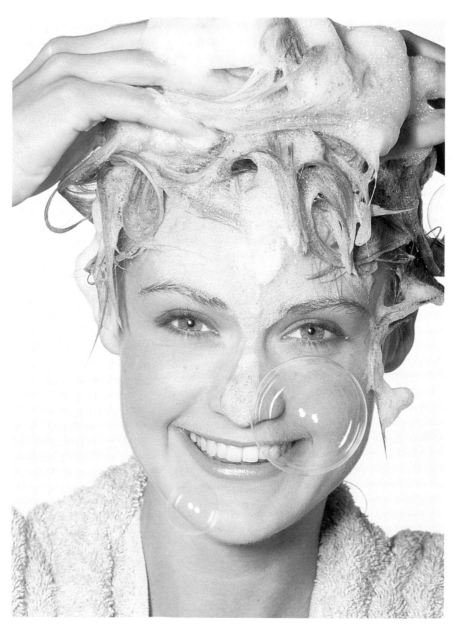

---

### Keep ahead of your hair

● A good cut is your hair's best friend, but after that it's up to you to keep it looking great with simple styling techniques.

● A daily shampoo and conditioning treatment will give your hair constant health and shine.

● A touch of mousse can control and transform any type of hair.

● A change of colour can perk up your looks and give your hair an exciting new dimension.

● A perm can lift fine, lank hair and allow for versatile styling.

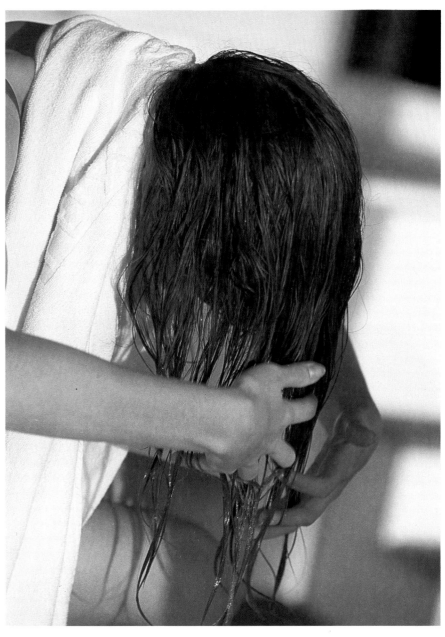

water as soapy, scummy water leaves deposits in the hair. Use a shower attachment for thorough rinsing.

Wet hair well with warm, never hot, water, then apply a small amount of shampoo from hand to hair, massaging it in gently with fingertips for a couple of minutes. Try to avoid massaging the length of hair as it causes tangles. If you shampoo daily you may only need one lathering up session before rinsing. Wet hair is vulnerable and less elastic so don't pull, tug or scrub or you'll break and damage the hair. Hair that feels squeaky is clean but the secret of really shiny hair is to rinse, rinse, and rinse again. You can never over-rinse.

## Conditioning

Shiny hair is a sign of hair in tip-top condition. If it's soft, shining and smooth to the touch, it can be one of your greatest assets.

The condition of your hair is naturally determined by the amount of moisture it contains. Shampooing hair doesn't dry it out, unless you use a harsh detergent like washing-up liquid; it puts water back into the hair, swelling the cuticles (the hair's surface outer layer). Conditioner locks moisture in and keeps the cuticle flat and smooth. The flatter hair lies (not on the head, but in each strand), the more it reflects light and the shinier it looks.

Hair can be roughened and dulled by overuse of hot curling tongs or rollers, misuse of hair driers, rough combs or hairbrushes, chemicals for bleaching, colouring and perming, elastic bands and even too much sun. Like skin moisturizers, conditioners protect hair from all elements.

Conditioning is important, whatever your hair type. Always use a conditioner after shampooing unless you prefer to use a styling

three days but with the upward swing towards health fitness and sports, the trend is for daily shampooing to keep hair looking its best.

Trial and error is the best method of deciding which shampoo agrees with your particular hair type. Often a shampoo for oily hair can be too harsh, causing split ends and stripping away natural oils (the faster oil is stripped away, the faster it is replaced, so some shampoos to combat oily hair don't necessarily help in the long term). Greasy hair tends to attract dirt so daily shampooing with a frequent-use shampoo, which is usually low-lather

*Never tug, scrub or pull hard on wet hair and use a spray attachment to rinse through thoroughly.*

and only needs one application, is the answer. Frequent hair washers often like to use baby shampoo, but this can, in fact, be harsh as it is formulated and tested to be milder on the eyes, not necessarily on the hair.

**How to shampoo**
How to shampoo your hair is important. Always comb or brush through your hair before shampooing. Never wash hair with bath

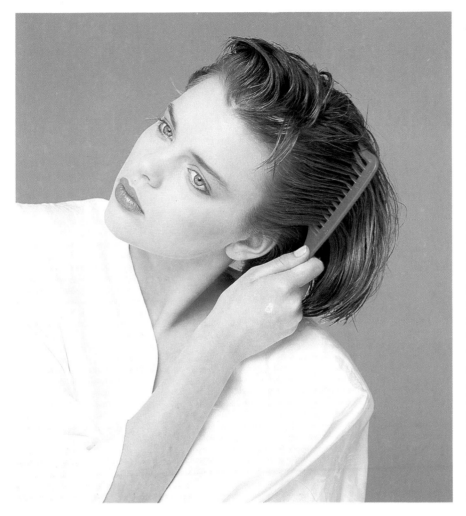

## Mousse

We've seen every imaginable gadget for hair styling, from tangle-free hair tongs to waffle-style crimpers. Now we're seeing something that you simply squeeze into the palm of your hand. With mousse you can tease your hair into almost any style and even add colour from dazzling damson to strawberry pink.

If you're nervous about using mousse, the foolproof technique is to squeeze just enough into the palm of one hand to fill an egg cup. Watch it expand for a few seconds to its full volume – sometimes twice or three times its original size – then rub the light, foamy mixture between your palms, and run it through your still-damp hair. Concentrate the mousse on the hair closest to the scalp; this is because hair has a natural preference to dry flat against the scalp, so to give it body you need to lift it away. If your hair feels sticky, you have used too much mousse. If your hair tends to be greasy don't choose a mousse with built-in conditioner.

Once the mousse is correctly applied, you can dry your hair by your usual method – hairdryer, setting it in rollers or letting it dry naturally.

**The effects of mousse** vary according to hair length. If your hair is long and curly, mousse will control the hair around the hairline, lifting it away from the scalp, and making the rest curlier.

If your hair is short and curly, mousse will add volume and encourage the curl. If your hair is short and straight, mousse will add more volume and hold a style in place if you use just a touch on towel-dried hair.

If your hair is cut into a one-length bob, it will probably be too heavy to benefit from mousse application, although it can be used sparingly to control flyaway ends.

mousse with built-in conditioning agents.

If your hair is fine and/or greasy, make sure you choose a conditioner with a light consistency. Flyaway hair with static electricity can be unmanageable so opt for a specifically formulated conditioner to take out the shocks. Split ends cannot be sealed by conditioners – they have to be cut off.

### How to condition hair
Pour conditioner into hands and gently rub into hair starting at the ends and working through gently. Leave for a minute or two and then rinse out thoroughly. (If your hair is greasy, you only need to condition the ends.) Comb through conditioner to detangle before thorough rinsing.

Particularly dry hair needs spec-

*Be sure to use a wide-toothed comb to take conditioner evenly and gently through the hair. Then rinse, rinse and rinse again.*

ific treatment. Rub henna wax or coconut oil/almond oil into the scalp. Cover head with a warm towel, cling-film or foil and leave for at least 15 minutes. Hair still has to be washed afterwards or the oils will leave the hair lank.

Today there are specific salon conditioning treatments which are readily absorbed by dry hair. All you need is heat, provided by hot lamps, driers or steamers.

Perms, highlighted or coloured hair should be given a regular treatment apart from conditioning. Many hairdressers offer treatments using natural ingredients, some tailor-made to hair type and colour.

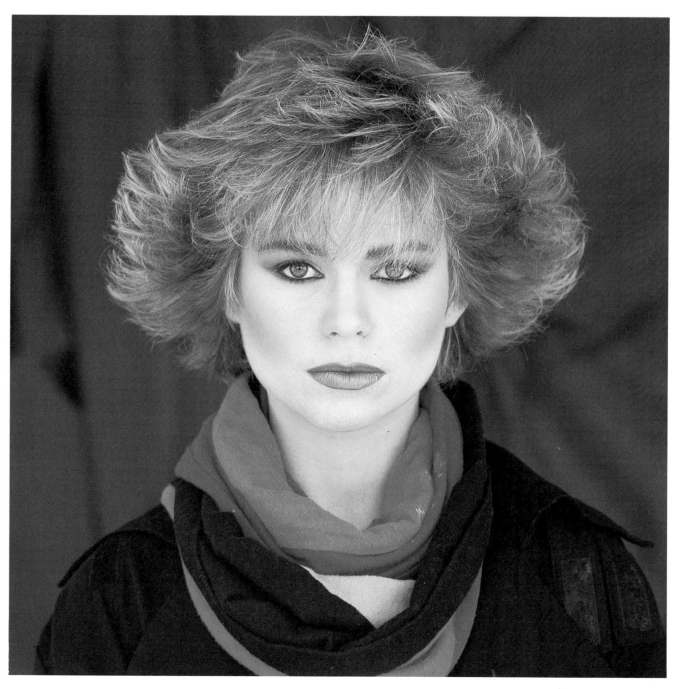

Mousse applied to dry hair has a stronger, longer-lasting effect; the water in towel-dried hair reduces the mousse's potency. So, if you feel you need more hold, your next experiment is to apply it to dry hair using the same method as for wet hair. Mousse can also be used to touch up a style in between washes. You can always brush it out and start again. Your hair may feel a little stiff but this is quite normal.

Long hair drawn up can benefit from a touch of mousse because (unlike hairspray, which puts a mantle around the hair), it helps the hair to support itself. The only problem is that it does attract dust and grime from the atmosphere so you may need to shampoo more frequently.

Hairdressers use mousse for exaggerated spiky short styles or simply to increase the hair's volume. They may dry the hair with head bent forward, applying mousse from the roots to the ends while drying.

*Mousse is the latest magic marvel for styling short hair – or adding volume to fine, flyaway hair.*

The only time when mousse should *not* be used is with heated curling tongs: the result is hard, brittle and over-heated hair.

## Styling aids

If you've become bored with your usual hairstyle try some of these gadgets and aids to achieve a bright new look.

106

**Bendy rollers** that look like long cigars are now available for curling up longer hair without using any heat. Made out of a synthetic fibre, rubber or cloth-padded, these 'sticks' are twisted round the hair in a way similar to the old 'rag' method. You can use on damp hair until dry or dry hair and leave for about 20 minutes or until the desired effect is achieved. To get a crinkled, wavy effect, twist hair first before winding it around. Try Molton Browners or Shumi Shophi-sticks.

**Styling airbrushes** are something to look out for. They act by blowing heat through the holes on the bar-rel. Use on damp hair to dry and curl at the same time.

**Setting gels** can slick back short hair and camouflage hair that needs washing in a matter of seconds. Some gels are ideal for the beach because they contain added protection factors against the sun's UV rays. They also safeguard hair against salt water and chlorine from swimming pools. Gels can also help to create wispy fringes and spiky effects.

*For full, wavy styles, like the one below, try bendy rollers and keep heated rollers for occasional use only.*

**Backcombing** fine hair may give it instant shape and style but the hair will droop and flatten later in the day. For extra lift and hold apply a mousse to dry hair and then back-comb with a narrow-toothed comb straight up from the front hairline.

**Heated rollers** are the answer if you are fed up with that classic bob. Use them to create a windswept look. For extra hold, use a setting lotion combed through dry hair. Leave a 2-in/5-cm panel of hair at the back straight – don't roller. Brush through with an air-vent brush for a really wild style.

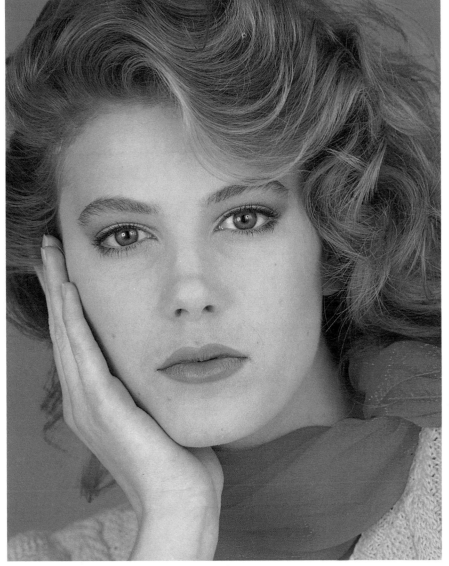

## Colouring

At some time in their lives most women have wanted to or actually have changed their hair colour and this has been going on for centuries; the ancient Romans and Greeks, for instance, used amazing dyes concocted from roots, leeches, dried flies and weird metallic substances to colour their hair.

Today's formulas are rather more versatile, offering a wide spectrum of colours to choose from. The woman with 'mousey' hair, for instance, is now a thing of the past – she's more likely to have sizzling blonde, warm brown or rich auburn hair. She is also being adventurous enough to change her hair colour to suit the season. And, when her hair starts to turn grey, she is refusing to let it age her, and is choosing from the mass of colourants on the market to banish dull grey hair.

### Hair structure and colour

As we know each strand of hair has three layers – the outer surface (cuticle); middle layer (cortex) and medulla (centre core). The cuticle is colourless and consists of fine scales – their degree of shine reflects the condition of the hair. The cortex gives hair its texture – coarse or fine. It also holds different layers of colour pigmentation. Different ratios of black, brown, red and yellow determine the natural colour of our hair.

## Types of colourants
There are three general types of colourant on the market – temporary, semi-permanent and permanent.

**Temporary colourants** give instant colour without permanent commitment. They won't lighten hair or penetrate the cortex, but simply coat the hair shaft. Temporary water rinses, setting lotions shampoos, gels, mousses and even sprays usually wash out after one shampoo. The colours may subtly tone down 'brassy' blondes or liven up brown and mousey hair with chestnuts and auburns. Fashionable temporary colours even offer gels you can streak through your hair with dazzlers like panache pink and ghastly green! And there are hair colour formulas that can be used like make-up. Finish your face, then 'mascara' on some liquid gold or copper around your fringe or wispy sides with a mascara-style wand. Colours can also be applied by means of hair sprays – which provide instant colour without having to wet hair and wash in.

**Semi-permanent colours** are usually lathered into wet hair so that they can penetrate the cuticle layer during developing time, only depositing a certain amount of colour in the cortex. They give a stronger colour change than the subtler temporaries but they cannot lighten hair since they do not strip away natural pigmentation. Semi-permanents are effective on mousey and light-brown hair but can also give brunettes rich auburn lights, and enhance grey hair. They normally last for up to 10 shampoos before fading out. Most manufacturers give detailed colour charts to determine which shade would work

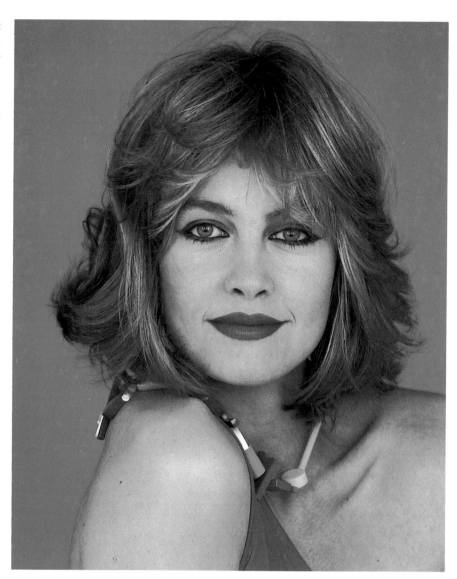

best for your hair colour and the time it takes for just a hint of highlights or a deeper shade. Some formulas designed to give extra colour and gloss are specially prepared for permed hair that has gone dull.

**Permanent colours** will lighten or darken, and won't wash out. These enter the middle layer of the hair (the cortex) and chemically alter its natural colour balance. They may fade just slightly but usually stay in until hair grows out. Its' wiser to go just a few shades lighter or darker to begin with since a drastic change of colour may make your complexion look sallow or too olive. The only problem with all-over permanent colouring is that you have root

**Above and right:** *There's nothing like a change of shade to boost your beauty morale. If you've never changed colour before, use a wash-in, wash-out rinse to see if you'll like the effect before taking the plunge with permanent colour.*

regrowth after four to five weeks. Professional salon tints should be retouched in the salon. But women are now tending to avoid overall colour changes and opting for tints and highlights or lowlights to give a more natural look.

## Colouring packs
Permanent colouring packs normally contain two bottles – a developer and a colour. With the darker reds and tawny browns, you

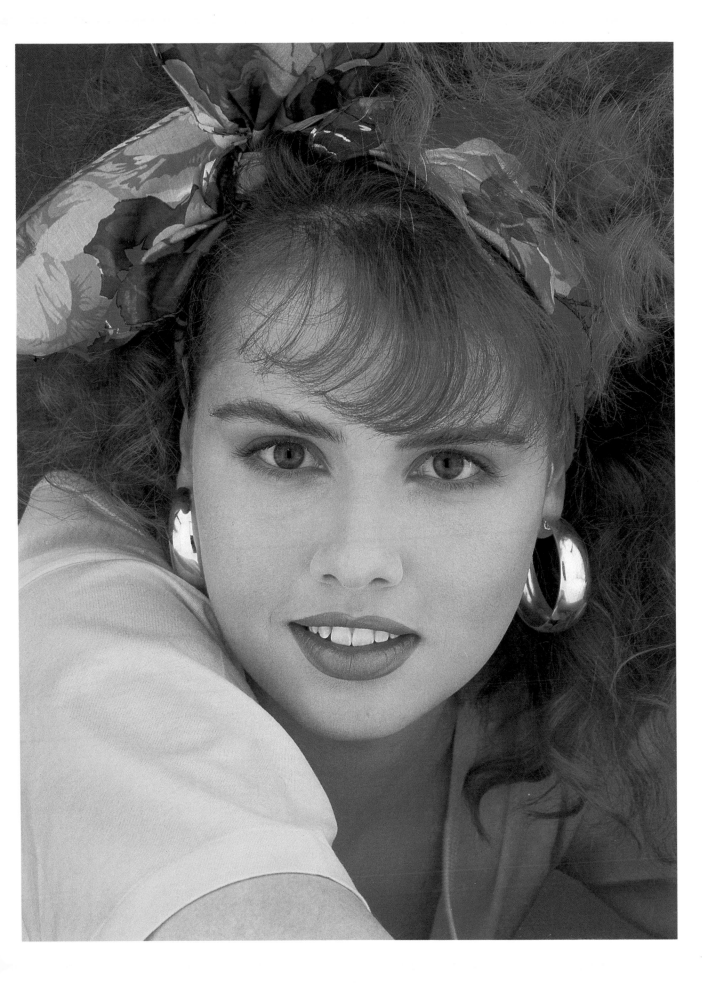

usually mix the two bottles together and use the mixture like a shampoo, rinsing out after the developing time. Don't rinse out before. Going blonde is slightly more complicated as you are not just adding tones, but replacing your hair's own natural colour. Blonde packs again contain two bottles – a lightener and a toner. The lightener, commonly peroxide or ammonia, strips the hair of natural colour. It also swells the middle layer so that when the second process of applying a toner or colour begins, the hair absorbs it. In retouching you have to concentrate on the roots first and then run colour through the rest of the hair for even coverage.

**Lighteners** are permanent bleaches. They don't add colour, they *remove* it. The more pigment that is removed, the lighter the hair becomes. Fair hair will lighten easily to a summer blonde but redheads won't go blonde easily. Home lightening kits, like the permanents, usually come with a toner and involve a two-stage process: first, colour is bleached out, then a toner is put in to cover brassiness or add different ranges of blonde from ash to honey. Bleached hair has to be retouched every four to five weeks. There are also lightening sprays on the market which you can use in the sun or with a hairdresser to give fair hair a summer-blonde lift.

**Highlights,** which are permanent, bleach the hair lighter in strands to give a shimmery effect. They don't add colour. They're great for giving a subtle lift to faded blonde and mousey hair. They can look flattering with older skin which lightens with age, particularly if the highlights are concentrated around the hairline and sides giving a softer, framing look. Once the strands of hair have been bleached it can still be coloured or toned to give a rich two-shaded effect. Highlights are best done professionally, either with the snug-fit-cap method where

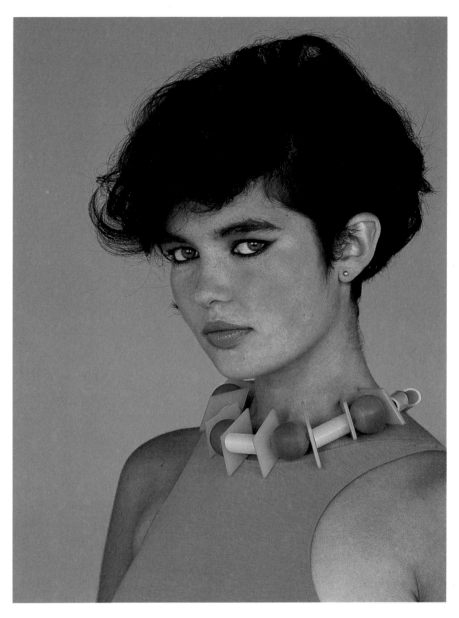

narrow strands are hooked through a holed hat, or the foil wrap method where bleached sections are rolled in metal foil. You can get hair streaking kits for home use which are easy to use if you just want to highlight your fringe but you may need a friend's help for the crown and back of head.

**Lowlights,** or permanent tints, are popular with brunettes. Reds, golds or both are blended into the hair to give a vibrant, shiny shimmer. Medium or dark brown hair looks great when rich claret or burgundy lights are added.

*Add an extra colour dimension to very dark hair with henna or a semi-permanent plum rinse.*

**Henna** is a natural vegetable dye – a finely crushed greenish powder prepared from an oriental shrub, *Lawsonia inermis alba*, containing red dye substances. It adds shining glossy red lights to black, red or brown hair but its lasting strength will depend on your hair texture. Don't use henna if your hair is fair or very grey – the result will be bright orange. The only problem with henna is that it builds up a conditioning coating on the hair so if you want to have a perm, always tell your hairdresser your hair is hennaed so that he or she will be able to work out the processing time for a successful body wave or curl. Some hennas contain metallic substances that won't work with a perm.

## Grey hair

Nearly everyone's hair goes grey with age but some people go grey when still in their teens, like top make-up artist Celia Hunter (see page 53). She didn't try to camouflage it because she preferred to make a feature of her extraordinary white/grey hair surrounding a very young face.

Pulling out grey hairs as they appear will not deter their growth. Genetics, hair types and textures and even stress can affect the hair's colour. A major shock could turn your hair white overnight. Normally, the greying process is a slow, gradual one, starting at the sides and temples. It can look distinguished in a man but is often ageing in a woman. Dark hair turned steely grey can look wonderfully effective. But for most of us the first signs of greying are less attractive and we want to conceal it.

If you're not happy with this process, you can resort to the latest colouring techniques (see below), or let nature take its course.

**Colouring grey hair** Grey hair can be ageing but there are some great cover-ups on the market. Remember as you get older your skin tones lighten so you should go for a colour just a shade lighter than your own natural colouring. And, your make-up should have a light touch, too. Hair that is totally grey and tinged with yellow (caused by the environment and smoking) can look dull. Fortunately there are water rinses, shampoos, toners and shaders with ash, oyster, silver or platinum tints which can lift out the yellow and give hair a shine. If you

are just beginning to go grey at the temples, you can have streaks put in the front professionally and then toned with a colour to give an even shimmer and camouflage the grey templed areas. Ask your hairdresser for advice. Colourants which contain chemicals can dry out the hair so it is best to give hair a once-a-month treatment pack, as well as conditioning after every shampoo.

## Pitfalls

A colour treatment and perm should never be carried out on the same day. Always leave a gap of a couple of weeks to let hair settle down after one chemical process. If you're going for a darker tint then it's best to have the perm first so that the perming chemicals don't lift out the colour.

Damage and disasters do happen. The most common problem for hairdressers is when hair has been bleached at home and chemically overprocessed, so that it dries out, turns brittle and snaps off. A good cut, conditioning treatment and toner is the answer. More difficult to correct is when hair has been permanently dyed a darker colour which won't lift. Whatever you try at home, make sure you carefully read the manufacturer's instructions and if you're not sure how your hair will react, snip off a small piece and do a test to see how it will look.

# Perming

Most of us have tried to put a little energy – curl, wave or body – into our hair, with heated rollers, tongs or just plain setting rollers. But the only way of making any kind of lasting curl is to have a perm.

## Development of the perm

More than 100 years ago the first permanent technique, the Marcel Wave was developed in France

whereby hot irons were used to kink the hair. This rather drastic-sounding technique was popular right through the 1920s. Shortages during the Second World War put a stop to perms, but with the return of prosperity, back came the electrically-heated perming clamp. Presumably women got tired of sitting under those heated gadgets for up to 10 hours because technology soon came up with an alternative – the cold wave. This system banished the hot rods in favour of a perming solution and neutralizer, which is more or less what is used today.

The bouffant hairstyles of the late Fifties and early Sixties put an end to perming for a while and were followed by the geometric cuts of the Sixties which relied on shiny, well-conditioned hair. So, for perming to make a comeback, the solutions needed to be kind to hair.

Perming made a comeback all right in the seventies. No sooner had we seen the soft, permed look than in came the hard 'wash 'n wear' curls that you can shampoo and leave to curl up naturally that Maria Schneider sported in the film *Last Tango in Paris*. And now of course, there's a perm to suit every hair type and lifestyle.

Scientists have developed perming techniques to cater for every fashion whim with the minimum of mess and fuss. All hair types, textures and lengths can be energized – bent into shape and moulded to suit.

There are new foaming waving lotions which don't drip; you simply aerosol on after you've rodded the hair. Some professional solutions for tinted hair can work in as little as five minutes and be neutralized in five minutes. Large perming rods without bands for natural perming are now commonplace. And the techniques are many and varied – you can roll or spiral-twist to achieve practically any style for any length of hair. And, once

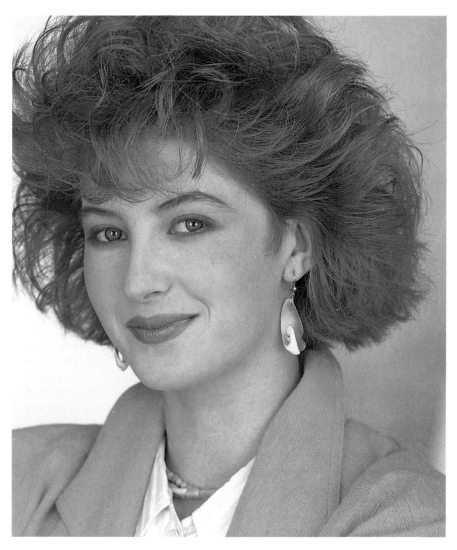

Those who are tempted to perm their hair at home should note that rectifying any damage done as a result of misuse keeps many hairdressers busy. For instance, if you wind your hair without first smoothing it over tissue paper and crinkling the ends around the rods, you will finish up with frizzed ends, and if you pull too tightly while rollering you will stretch vulnerable hair that has been broken down chemically so that when it's unwound you may find crinkles, band marks and breakage.

Before embarking on a perm, seek professional advice. You may simply need your hair layered, cut or coloured to give it lift. If your hair is dry or brittle your hairdresser may advise you not to perm it.

### Perm-ability

**Lank/greasy hair** will benefit from a perm because it dries it out slightly and gives it more bounce.

**Fine flyaway hair** can be the most difficult hair to perm.

**Coarse, wiry hair** tends not to perm well because its dry, porous nature makes it retain solutions quickly, often leaving hair brittle. Soft, gentle perming and masses of conditioner are needed.

**Grey hair** is also porous and can be difficult to perm since there are two hair types – grey and natural. A hairdresser can look at the percentage of grey and advise on how an even result can be achieved.

**Naturally wavy hair** tends to be stronger at the bottom edges, nape of neck and ears so you could benefit from a top-of-head perm only if you have a flat crown.

you've got a perm you can make your hair full of body or bounce, or dried with mousse you can achieve that untamed look.

### The perming process

Hair is made up of the three layers: the cuticle, the cortex and the medulla. The cortex, the middle layer, made up of tiny cells that link into chains, determines the hair's strength and colour. The pattern of these chains varies depending on the amount of natural wave or curl in the hair.

The perming solution soaks through the cuticle into this second layer and loosens the chain links so that they reform and mould together into shape controlled by the perm rods. This is followed by the

*Know your hair type before you consider a perm (see chart on right).*

neutralizing process which stops further development and seals the hair shape. The final hair shape will be determined by how long the perming solution is left on.

### Curl or body wave?

It is the way hair is cut, layered and, more important, the method and size of rods used on the hair that will determine whether you end up with a body wave or extra curl. Generally, the larger the rods, the softer the perm. Fine, layered hair works well permed and even long, fine hair can be spiral wound to give rippling waves or curls – ideal for wash 'n' wear looks.

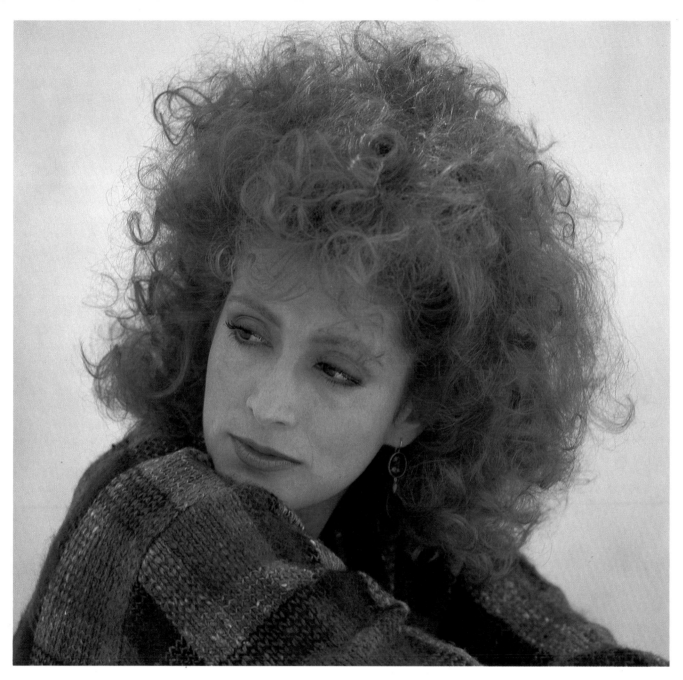

**Points for success** If you are going ahead with a home perm, take note of the following:

● Analyze your hair type and if you are not sure, ask a friend whether she thinks your hair is fine, coarse, thick or lank.

● Choose a perm specially formulated for the effect you want, such as curls or soft waves.

● Read the instructions carefully and be guided by the test-curl method.

● Get a friend to help you to wind the roots at the back of your head in the right tension and evenness.

● Small rods give tighter curls; use larger rods for soft curls.

● Split ends will frizz. Have them trimmed off beforehand or, if you want your hair reshaped, get a professional cut first, remembering that perming gives a shorter look.

● Don't home-perm hennaed, colour-treated, streaked, highlighted or partially grey hair because the perming solution works faster on the colour-treated or grey hair, giving an uneven result. A hairdresser will feel the different textures of

*Before tackling a home perm, seek professional advice to make sure your hair's in good shape.*

your hair and judge how much perming it can take.

● Don't perm on already permed hair.

● Never attempt to perm very long hair.

● Always, always use a conditioner after shampooing and a regular treatment pack once your hair is permed to keep it healthy.

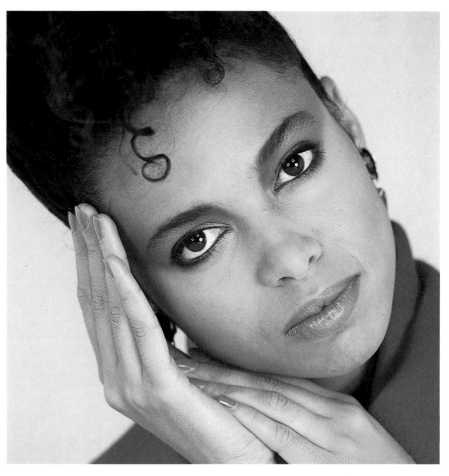

## Afro hair

*New techniques have made styling Afro hair much easier and more versatile.*

Styling has come a long way for Afro hair since the black-is-beautiful look of the Sixties. New trends in Afro fashion offer far greater flexibility, exploiting the hair's natural assets rather than trying to straighten it into more European styles. Braiding, plaiting and sewing in extensions (which can be shampooed and conditioned without unbraiding) have outclassed the beaded look. The new versatility in Afro hairdressing has been made possible by clever cutting, moulding, perming and colouring techniques. Layered cuts and relaxing perms can reshape hair and colours can emphasize hair shape.

### Cuts

Clipper cuts at the sides show off high cheekbones and features. Razor cuts give fringes a spiky look. Sculptured cuts, when the hair is moulded closer to the head, not only look fabulous (think of Grace Jones) but are very practical for sportswomen.

### Perms

Perming usually involves relaxing tightly frizzed hair by means of a chemical perming process to remove the kinks. The result can be either straight hair or a looser curl such as the spiral or corkscrew curl. Perming is good for most Afro hair types – unless hair is in very bad condition.

Afro hair can be fine, frizzy and difficult to perm, as can fine, fly-away European hair. Coarse textured hair also resists perming and may need several test strengths before all-over perming. Afro hair, unlike European hair, may need perming more frequently on the roots since the tight and curly root regrowth combined with the more loosely curled ends may be difficult to comb or tong into any style.

### Colouring

Colour can emphasize the shape and cut of Afro hair. Temporary spray-on colours in rich mahogany or pinks, reds, lilacs and even blues can liven up the sides and the hairline. Sculptured Afro hair can also take daring zig-zag colour shapes for a really dramatic look.

Colour baths work like a semi-permanent hair colour to brighten up dull hair, washing out after six to eight shampoos, without colour build-up. Tints and bleached highlights can also look stunning on the front or sides or run through the hair – depending on how many chemical processes your hair has already undergone and whether it can stand the extra pressure without snapping.

Dry scalps can result from using too many harsh chemicals. Massage an oil into scalp and roots; almond, coconut, jojoba or simply olive oil will all provide a suitable treatment. Wrap a hot wet towel to steam or wind around cling-film or foil to heat in the treatment.

### Shampoos and conditioners

It is important for Afro hair to keep in moisture. So shampoos should be low-lather, mild formulas followed by easy-to-rinse-through conditioners. Conditioning treatments should be based on oil rather than petroleum or vaseline which tend to clog up the scalp and block pores.

### Mousses and gels

Styling foam mousses with added conditioners like jojoba and milk oils give Afro hair a shine. Leave them in for extra hold. Gels slicked into the hair give it extra sheen and some have wash-out fun, crazy colours. Aerosol shiny sprays also add extra lustre.

# Massaging your scalp

If you sometimes hate your hair the answer may well be in your own hands. Stimulating the scalp with your fingers increases its circulation, flexibility and health. Your hair will benefit by showing a new shine and oil control.

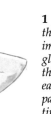

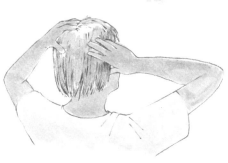

**1** *The large muscles that run up the sides of the head from ear to crown are often tight, impeding the balance of the sebaceous glands. Loosen them up like this: anchor thumbs behind your ears; place fingers above ears and move scalp in small circles with pads of fingers. Keep moving up an inch at a time and repeat massage circles up to crown.*

**2** *Work on the back of the head by circling with the finger pads of one hand and moving from base of skull to crown. Work on section behind ear, then centre back. Change hands to do the other side of head.*

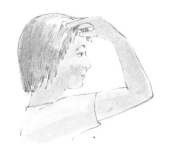

**3** *The front and crown part of the scalp is often so rigid that it can lead to lack of nourishment and thinning hair in front. Circle all over the area, but always take care to use soft finger pads . . . never nails.*

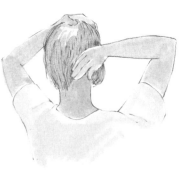

**4** *While you're working to relax your scalp don't forget the tension-prone tendons and muscles at back of neck. Pinch (gently) between fingers and thumb. Work from base of skull and across from ear to ear.*

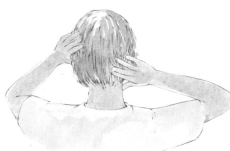

**5** *Whenever tension ties up the muscles, the circulation no longer flows freely. The back hairline is a prime target. Release the area by pressing lightly with fingertips all round the base of the skull.*

# Dandruff

Dandruff is just a build-up of dead skin cells. It is not catching. The result of a speed-up in cell turnover, it is thought to be caused by a chemical change in the body, probably associated with stress, poor eating habits and wrong usage of hair products.

The Philip Kingsley Trichological Clinic, in London and New York, estimates that 75 per cent of city dwellers have dandruff. It strikes everyone at one time or another. Just how severe your problem is depends on the rate at which your cell turnover has speeded up. We normally renew and shed our skin cells every 28 days, but a person with dandruff is shedding faster than this.

There are two types of dandruff: oily and dry. Most dandruff sufferers come into the oily category, which means they're not shedding on their shoulders (dandruff isn't visible on their clothes) – it stays in their hair. Those with dry dandruff, on the other hand, will have a snowy collar.

**How to combat dandruff**
Try an anti-dandruff shampoo. Most contain zinc omadine or pyruthione, said to suppress cell turnover. If they don't work (and they often don't), try daily shampooing (one wash only) with a mild, not a dandruff, shampoo.

After shampooing, comb your hair, (keep brushes and combs immaculate). Then dab on a scalp lotion made with one part mouthwash and two parts camphor water.

Cut down on sugary and fatty foods, especially cheese. Eat lots of fresh fruit and vegetables. And do your best to cut down the stress in your life and relax. Because, as Philip Kingsley says in *The Complete Hair Book*, 'In its own peculiar way, dandruff is nature's way of telling you to slow down, back off, calm

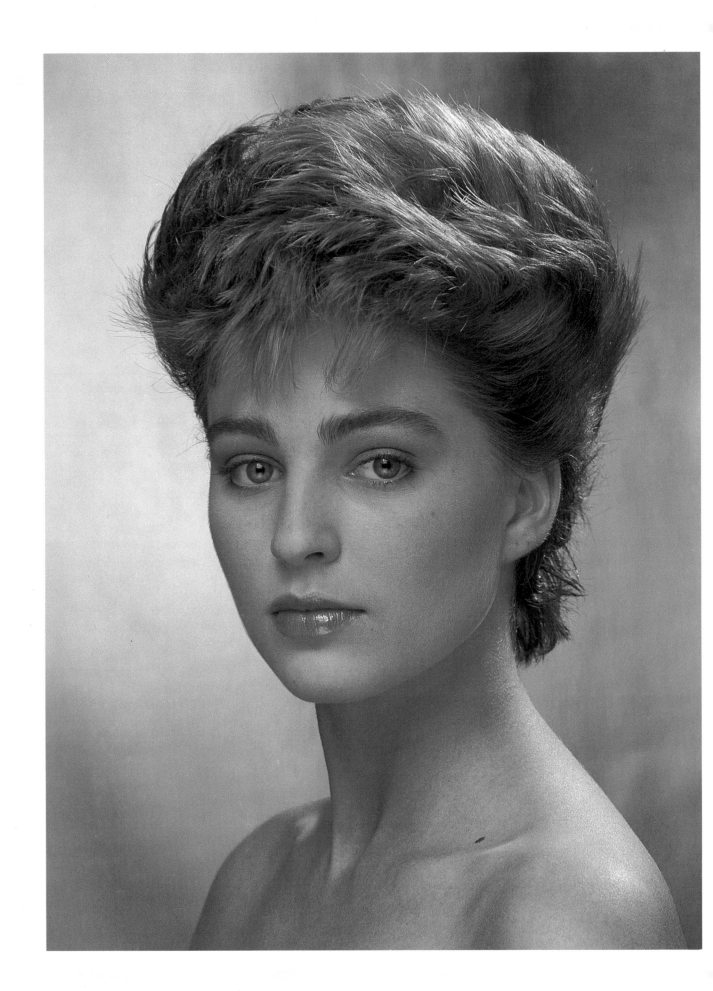

down.' If your problem persists, consult a trichologist.

## Philip Kingsley's winter pick-me-up

Take two eggs, the juice of one lemon, two half eggshells of witch-hazel, one half eggshell of safflower oil. Mix together, then apply with cotton-wool ball to scalp and whole length of hair. Cover with shower hat and leave for 30 minutes. Remove shower hat, massage for 10 minutes, then rinse. Finally, shampoo and condition as usual.

## Expert help

Trichologists are trained to recognize and treat hair and scalp problems. To find one in your area, write, enclosing a stamped, self-addressed envelope, to the Institute of Trichologists, 228 Stockwell Road, London SW9 9SU.

# Hair loss

So busy are we lavishing care and attention on the hair we see, we tend to forget the very important living section that's hidden away under the scalp. Once a hair pops through the scalp, it's nothing but a dead protein substance, similar to your nails or the hooves and horns of animals.

## Moulting

There's no need to start having fits if your hair comes out in handfuls. A normal healthy adult head loses 80-100 hairs a day – often more in spring and autumn when we tend to go into a big moult, just like furry animals. With around 100,000 hairs left on show, you can relax, unless you're suffering from a genuine thinning thatch (very unusual in a woman) in which case you should seek medical advice.

*Shiny, healthy hair depends on a good, varied diet – and the sensible use of the right equipment.*

When a hair gets to the end of its growth phase, it falls out and the follicle then takes a break for a few months before going into production again. Some people have a longer hair life cycle than others, so it's no good pining for hair you can sit on if yours has a struggle to make it to shoulder length – just accept your genetic inheritance.

## Keep calm

A major operation, illness, emotional shock, stress, certain drugs or a hormonal upheaval can all cause a heavier hair loss than normal as well as slowing down regrowth, but don't panic; your hair will recover, shortly after your body does. Worrying about hair loss is counter-productive; the more you worry, the more you accentuate the problem.

If your hair is looking tatty and you decide to have the ends trimmed, it will immediately appear thicker and healthier. Although contrary to popular belief, cutting does not encourage a faster, more luxuriant growth of hair; it simply gets rid of split, thin ends, making the remainder look more abundant.

Unless they are trimmed off, split ends will eventually work right up the hair shaft.

---

## Points to remember

**Brushing** your hair 100 times a day does not give you a 'crowning glory' – it heats up your hair and scalp and dries out valuable moisture.

**Bristle brushes** aren't necessarily better than plastic ones – it depends on your hair texture. For coarse, thick hair, brushes with wide gaps between teeth or bristles are most suitable as hair slips through easily without tugging.

**Vigorous towel drying** can cause too many tangles and friction. Wrap a towel around your head, turban style, for a few minutes, letting it blot up excess water naturally.

**A wide-toothed comb** is kinder than a brush when de-tangling wet hair. Comb from ends, gradually working up to scalp.

**Any hot appliance** – such as tongs, rollers, driers – can dry out hair if over-used.

**Sun** damages hair. Ultra-violet rays in the sun can dry, bleach, and increase the porous quality of your hair. If you have a headful of chemical processing such as a perm, bleach or tint, then protect your hair with a hat, scarf or protection lotion or gel.

Fine, flyaway hair can be a flop by the sea so add a mousse or light hairspray to your luggage. Try to give hair a holiday and leave behind your heavy heat equipment – try mousse and finger drying for a more relaxed style. If you want to brighten up your hair to go with your suntan, try using a fun-coloured gel for streaking in and giving hair a holiday lift.

**All chemical processing** dries out hair so go carefully on the after-styling with rollers and tongs and always, always, use a heavier-duty conditioner.

# Celebrity Style

*Every beautiful princess, every genuine superstar, every stunning celebrity and top cover girl has appeared in* Woman's Own *over the years. Here some of our favourites share their beauty secrets with you. Each one is exceptional in her own way. What they have in common are attributes any woman needs to be truly attractive: a warm personality, a zest for life and the determination to make the best of themselves.*

*Isabella Rossellini*

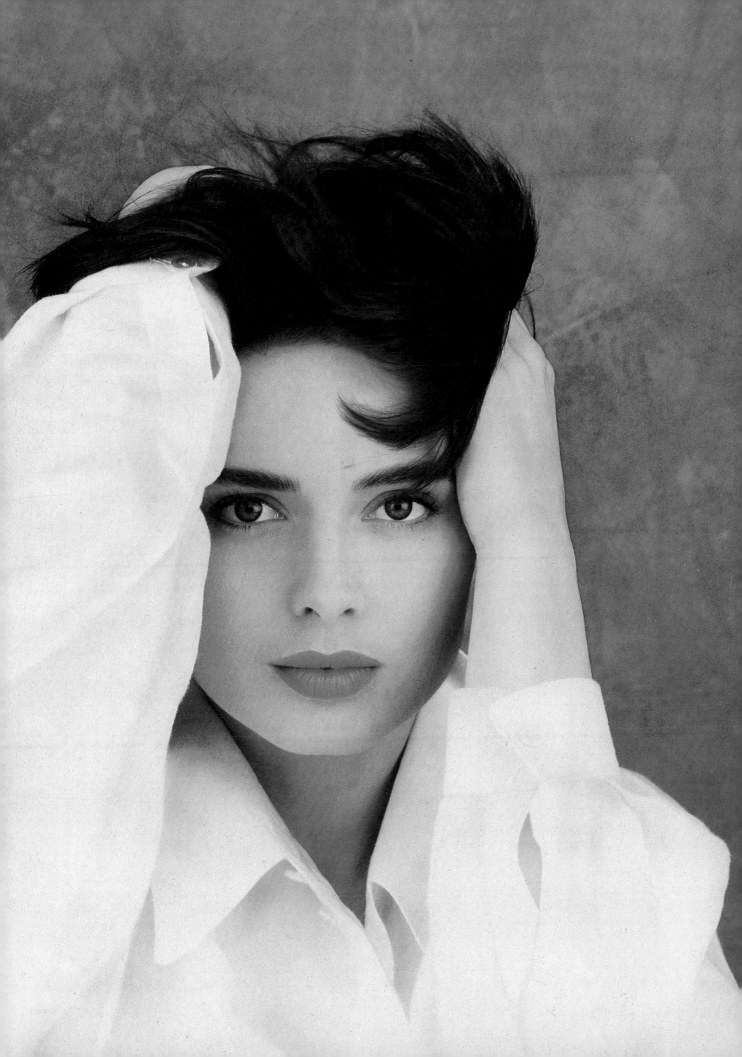

## Isabella Rossellini

At 30, an age when most models would be hunting for the anti-wrinkle cream, Isabella Rossellini won a million-dollar contract to promote Lancôme cosmetics (see page 119). Two years later, in 1985, she made her international film début, co-starring with Mikhail Baryshnikov in *White Nights*.

Isabella's warm wonderful smile and wide expressive eyes are inherited from her mother, the late Ingrid Bergman, and her dark Latin looks from her father, film director Roberto Rossellini.

### Sensible diet

She lives with her daughter Elettra in New York but, unlike millions of other New Yorkers, doesn't believe she needs to jog and swallow masses of vitamins to stay healthy. 'I don't jog because there's no grass where I live and it isn't good to run on concrete. I don't take vitamins regularly because it you eat properly there's no need. I suppose it's my European background but I don't

like canned or frozen foods. I prefer to shop every day for fresh food. I have fruit juice and toast for breakfast. At lunchtime, I like pasta – it's not so fattening if you just have it with a light tomato sauce – and then I have fish or meat, salad and cheese in the evening. I enjoy wine with my dinner. For exercise I like swimming and I also belong to a gym. I try to go at least once a week – more if I'm not working.'

### Hair and skin care

She keeps her hair short 'because it stays healthier that way. I wash and condition it every morning. It's important to keep my skin good so each week I use a mask – sometimes a cleansing mask or Lancôme's Masque 10 which reduces puffiness under the eyes – very important for me if I have to be up extra-early for photos. I use moisturizer every day and a special eye cream. At night, I use a slightly richer cream. If I've been working constantly for some time, then every four weeks I go for a professional facial. It's my favourite beauty treat because the end result is so dramatic!'

## Chris Evert Lloyd

One of tennis's greatest-ever champions, Chris Evert Lloyd is also one of its most attractive ambassadors. She appears beautifully groomed and has an enviably trim figure. But she's modest about her looks.

'I know my faults. Beauty is a state of mind, however. I was a celebrity at 16, with all the problems that came with it. Today, I have confidence and a very happy private life.'

### Diet and exercise

She credits husband John with the successful diet and exercise plan that keeps her in such good shape. 'I was eating too much fat and protein for an athlete . . . the simpler the carbohydrate the faster it works into your system. I used to eat eggs and pancakes for breakfast, but now it's natural cereal with bran, a banana and fruit juice. At lunch I have a sandwich, something like turkey or cheese with lettuce on wholewheat bread, plus a piece of fruit and my one treat of the day – a can of Tab.

'In the evening we always enjoy a big meal – often chicken cooked on the barbecue, with a baked potato, vegetables and a huge salad. I might have something like a bowl of strawberries for dessert. The only time I go crazy on desserts is when we're in England – John's mum makes marvellous puddings! I enjoy white wine but there's something about my system that makes it react really fast, so two glasses is my limit.'

Chris finds that a month off from tennis means she can put on weight easily, so 'both John and I do aerobics four or five times a week. I do stretching exercises before each match – for flexibility and to prevent the possibility of injuries. Your back and legs can take a tremendous pounding if you're playing on concrete for three hours. If I have a

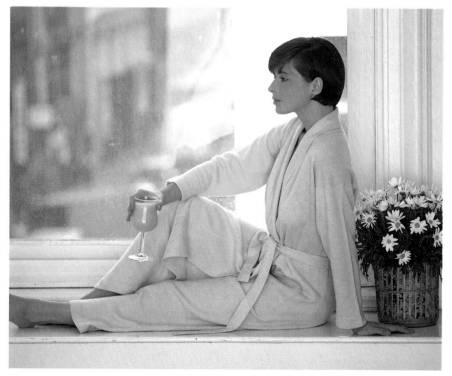

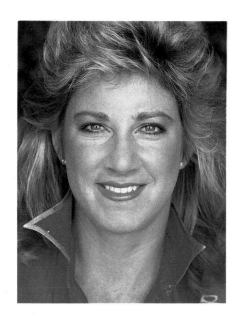

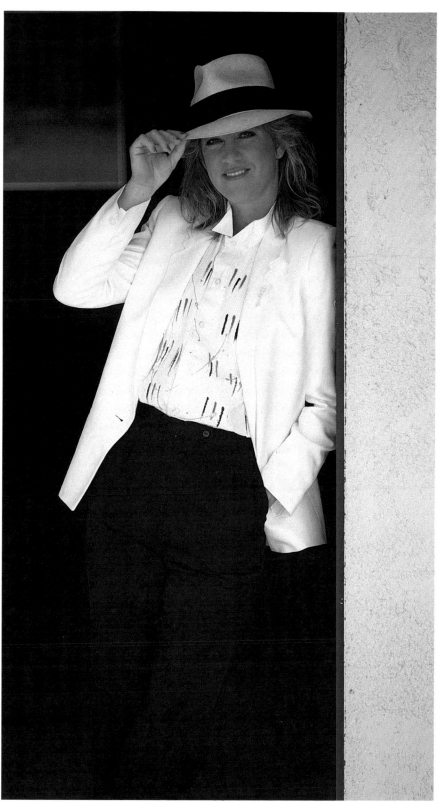

week off, I also try to work out with weights at a gym to strengthen my arms and upper body. Wherever I am I have to have nine hours' sleep. If I can't be in bed by midnight and sleep till nine, the next day is shot for me.'

The Lloyds have four main bases and, wherever they are, Chris always heads for the nearest masseuse. 'It's my greatest luxury. Of course, it's necessary for an athlete after a match; but to me it's the biggest treat money can buy, too.'

## Beauty tips

Travelling all the time, and having to cope with constant changes of water, can cause her skin to break out. 'For the past couple of years, though, I've been following a skin-care routine, using natural-based products. First I wipe my face over with a hot flannel, then wash with a natural glycerine soap, rinse well and clean again with rose-water freshener. That's followed with a spray mist before I apply an aloe-based cream. I cleanse the same way at night, followed by a night cream. Once a week I use either a honey-and-almond scrub or a clay mask. It sounds like a lot of work, but I'm really interested in the way I'll look at 40 – especially after practically living in the sun!

'I like to have a tan but I'm careful. I wear sunglasses whenever possible and never sunbathe without covering my face with a sun hat or towel. My hair's thin and fine so it can't take too much back-combing or hot rollers to give it style. I wash and condition it every day and have it trimmed and highlighted every two months: wherever I am, I've got the name of a hairdresser who can cope with it!'

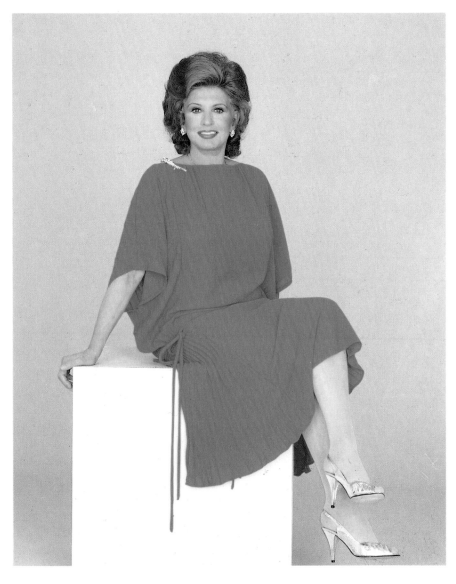

## Patricia Phoenix

For more than 20 years, she was the red-headed temptress of The Rover's Return. Pat Phoenix left *Coronation Street* in 1983 but she – and her career – are still going strong. At 62, she has a glamorous aura and incredible vitality. She is surprisingly petite, but with incredibly long, shapely legs. 'I always say God gave me good legs and forgot about the rest of me,' she laughs. 'I'm very short-waisted and if I don't watch my weight I can look incredibly dumpy.'

Before any stage tour or new TV series, she tends to go on a strict diet. 'It's a question of discipline – and avoiding fattening snacks during rehearsals.'

### Beauty routine

She says she doesn't have time for a complicated beauty routine, 'but I do have one cream I wouldn't be without. It's a mixture of honey, beeswax and ginseng which I use for everything – cleansing and moisturizing. That's the extent of my skin care but I'd never dream of going out without make-up and my hair done because I don't want to let my fans down.'

## Jane Seymour

Jane Seymour was born Joyce Frankenburg but chose Henry VIII's third wife's name for her acting career because she was the one who didn't get her head chopped off! Just as well because Jane's head has turned out to be her fortune. 'I've always had long hair, and it's me – I can't imagine having a short style,' she says. At home, Jane has a quick and simple routine for hair care. 'I shampoo first thing in the morning under the shower. I use a mild shampoo, plus a wide-toothed comb to run through a light conditioner. Whenever possible, I let my hair dry naturally and then go through it gently with a bristle hair brush. I have a trim every six weeks or so to keep the ends healthy.'

### Exercise and beauty

Married to David Flynn, an American film producer, Jane has two children, Katie and Sean. She kept in shape during her pregnancies with the Jane Fonda exercise routine five times a week. 'To be honest, I didn't have time to do any exercises afterwards, I was too busy breast-feeding on demand around the clock!'

During filming for the starring role in the *Winds of Remembrance*, the sequel to *Winds of War*, despite hot lights and heavy film make-up, Jane's skin stayed immaculate. 'I always make sure it's clean. For really deep cleansing I steam my face with a hot flannel to open the pores, then use a honey and almond scrub. I like toners without alcohol because my skin is slightly sensitive. My main beauty "must" is a light fluffy collagen mousse which I keep in the fridge.'

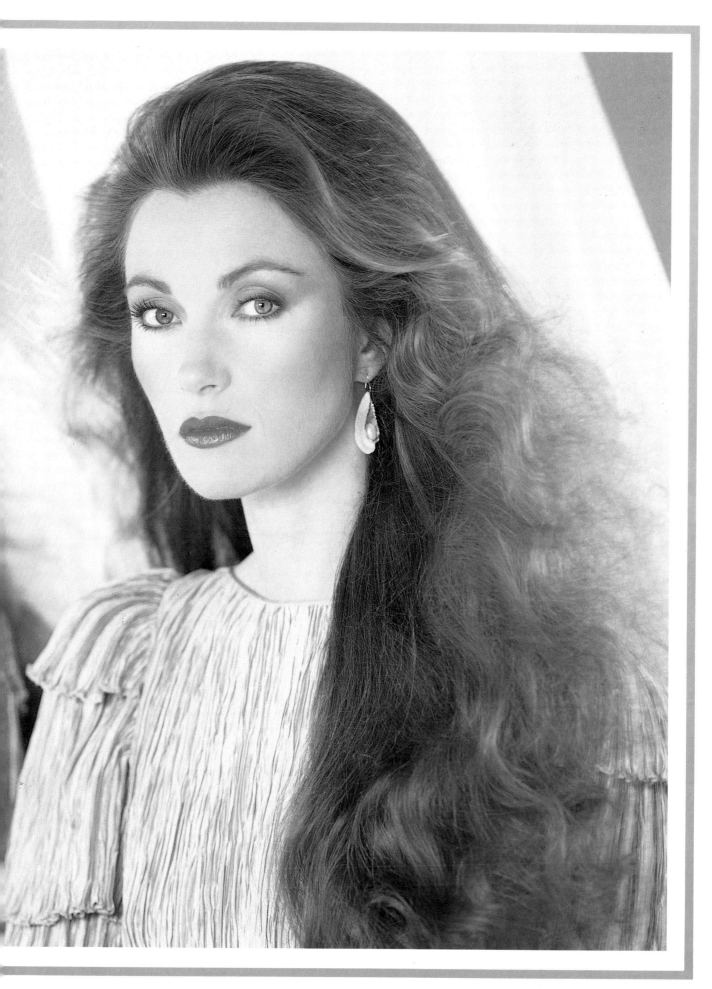

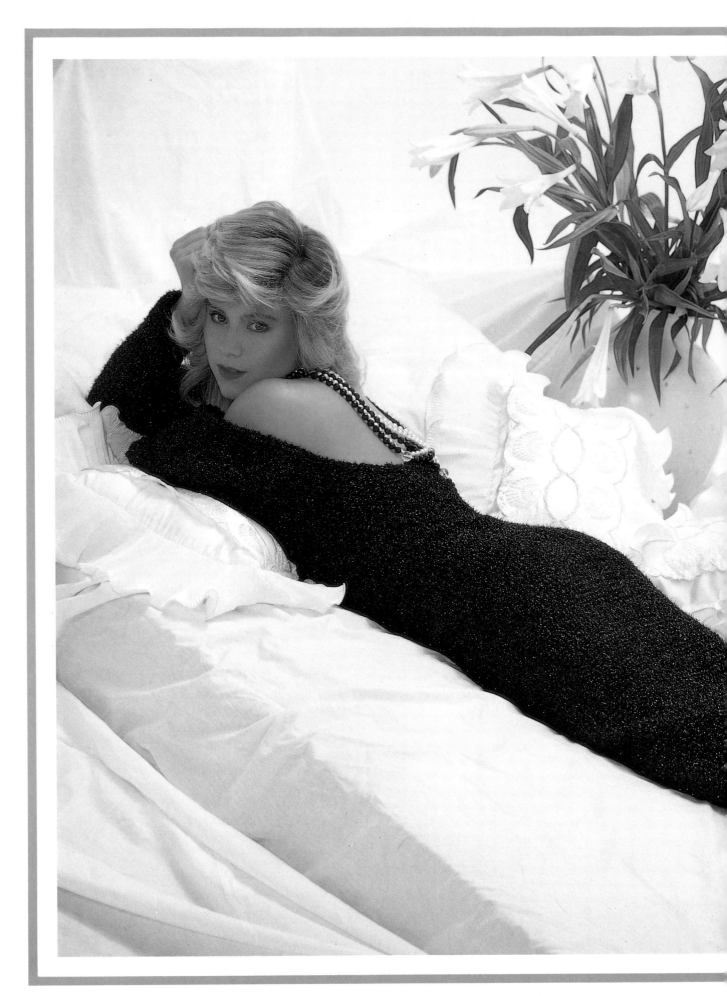

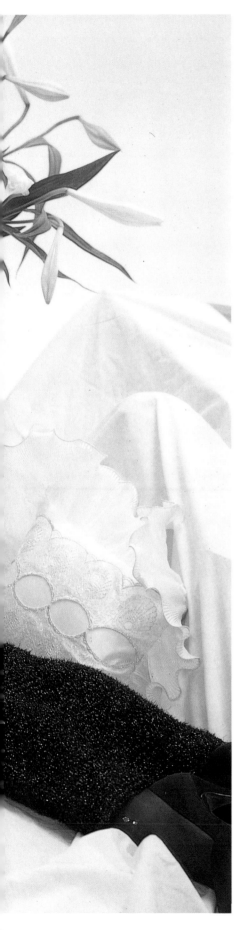

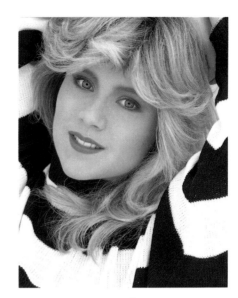

## Samantha Fox

At 16, Samantha Fox won a newspaper model contest. Just a few years later, she's a fully-fledged celebrity, spending more time appearing on chat shows, opening discos and making records than she does posing for glamour photographs.

'I inherited me shape from me gran,' Samantha explains. 'People think I must do special exercises to keep my boobs firm but I don't. I like swimming because it's an all-round body-toner and I'd like to say I work out regularly at a gym but, to be honest, I don't because I don't have the time. I love dancing, though, and that helps to keep me fit. When I'm out, I enjoy a bottle of bubbly now and again but mostly I drink spritzers (white wine and soda water). They're not fattening and a couple can last you all evening. I don't consciously diet – I love fish and chips and McDonalds hamburgers but I don't go mad. I believe in eating a bit of everything in moderation.'

Just before her visit to Australia, in the summer of 1986, she said 'a magazine there voted me cover personality of the year and I'll be doing cover shoots and appearing on the telly and, I hope, getting a good suntan.'

### Skin care

Sam has flawless skin and keeps it looking smooth by applying a rich, moisturizing body lotion for dry skin (Revlon) all over after every bath or shower. 'I either shave my legs or use a hair removing cream.'

Her face is quite sensitive. 'In my business, we have to wear a lot of make-up and seem to be forever taking it off and putting it on, so I use a mild range of cleansing preparations from Marks and Spencer. I also like their eye make-up remover cream. I can't stand those oily pads!' Whenever possible, Samantha goes without make-up to give her skin a rest, 'but I'd never go out without mascara – I'd feel bald!'

### Best dressed head

Bald she certainly isn't – in fact her hair was voted Best Dressed Head by The British National Federation of Hairdressing. 'It's fine but there's a lot of it,' says Samantha. 'I have it streaked and lightly permed. I wash it every day with a mild shampoo, followed by conditioner. When I'm not working I leave it to dry naturally to give it a rest from the heated rollers and backcombing.'

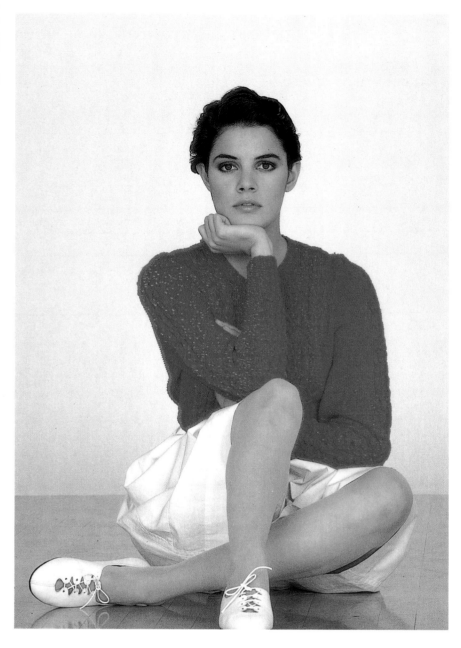

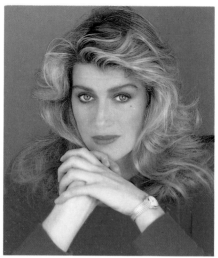

## Selina Scott

One of Britain's most professional TV personalities, Selina Scott also rates as one of the nicest. She posed unflinchingly for more than an hour in a grey drizzle and biting wind for this picture. 'The most appealing asset any woman can have is good skin. Its beauty is immediately apparent, it enhances her eyes, her hair – everything. It's worth going to some lengths to maintain it and if you're lucky enough to be born with good skin, it's worth protecting.'

'I love to see a very old woman, of, say, 80 or 90, with lovely skin. The kind that has never seen the cosmetic surgeon's knife and known only simple, but regular care.

### Fresh air and water
'I try to get as much fresh air as possible. Ideally I would walk briskly for 30 minutes every day. It helps that I live near Hyde Park.

'Water is my other beauty ally. Long before it was bottled in the UK, I used to collect rainwater in a barrel to use on my face. I drink half a pint of sparkling mineral water when I wake each morning and continue throughout the day. I suppose I reach around six glasses. I never drink London tap water so I buy a lot of bottled water.

## Tahnee Welch

In 1985, one of the top box office hits in the USA was a gentle comedy called *Cocoon* starring Tahnee Welch. This young actress's dark yet delicate looks are somehow familiar . . . her mother is Raquel Welch. The second-generation Welch worked as a model to pay her acting school fees before becoming an actress.

She does not, however, ascribe to the old glamour Hollywood tradition. 'I tend to live in baggy pants and man-size T-shirts and I love over-sized jackets. I don't possess any dressy clothes, but if I'm going out for the evening I make myself look special by using more eye make-up, a strong lip colour and a wilder-looking hairstyle.' Her biggest beauty plus is yoga – taught her by Raquel – which means she stays calm in the most frantic film-set situation.

'I eat all kinds of food, but my first love is fruit; grapes, bananas, whatever is in season. I also try to include a little butter in my diet each day – I'm convinced it improves my complexion.

## Sleep

'When I was doing Breakfast Television, I'd get around two hours sleep during the night (I catnapped during the day) and always on waking, I splashed my face with cold water. I use a moisturizer, but have only once indulged in a facial. The beauty salon is really unknown to me.

'When I do get a straight eight hours' sleep, I can see the difference immediately in my skin and I certainly believe that, along with fresh air, sleep ranks highly.

'I'd never take a lot of sun on my face because I think it's harmful to sensitive skin like mine, but I do suntan my body. It's the least of my priorities, however, but a light suntan is very appealing.'

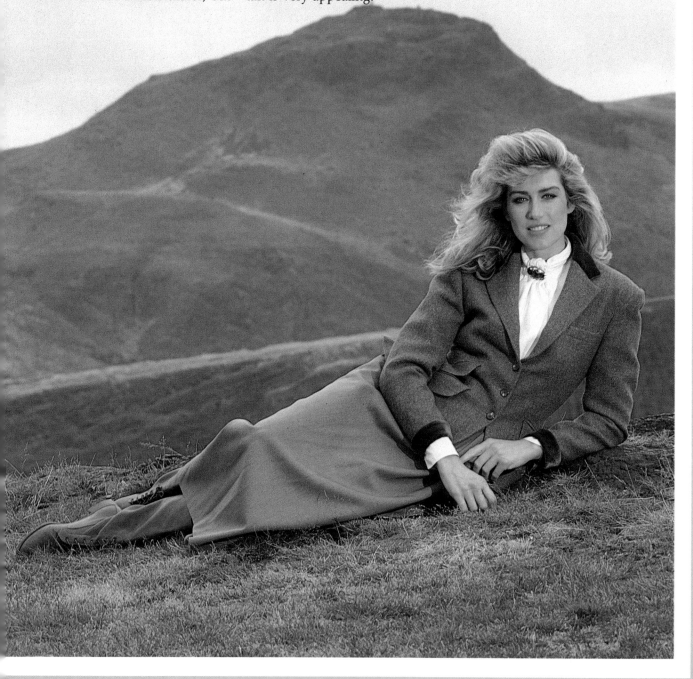

# Joan Collins

She is, without a doubt, a pheno-menon. Incredibly rich, incredibly beautiful and incredibly successful – and she works incredibly hard to ensure she stays that way

Apart from *Dynasty*, she has a lucrative contract to promote per-fume, her own range of sunglasses and her own production company, run by husband Peter Holm, to make mini-series and films dur-ing her summer break from being Alexis. 'It takes a lot of hard work to keep all the projects going – but luckily I'm blessed with a lot of energy and *joie de vivre*. My biggest luxury is time to myself. If ever I get the chance I relax with my feet up on the bed, reading magazines or watching TV. If it's warm enough I lie by the pool and sunbathe. I never expose my face to the sun, however.'

## Make-up

Off-screen, the thick foundation necessary for the hot *Dynasty* life is replaced with a light make-up base – Clinique is her favourite brand – and even when she's working she prefers to do her own make-up.

'I don't like other people doing it because they pull the skin. I use good old Nivea to take off my make-up and I'll go for any moisturizer around – most of the major com-panies have good ranges. But I always swap them around because the skin can get used to one product. I love Christian Dior mascara because you can wash it off with water. I don't like oil-based remov-ers because they can leave the eyes looking puffy the next morning, which is no good in my job.'

She is often up by 5a.m. and manages to fit in a 15-minute work-out session at a gym three times a week before going to work.

## Travelling in comfort

When she's not on set, she spends

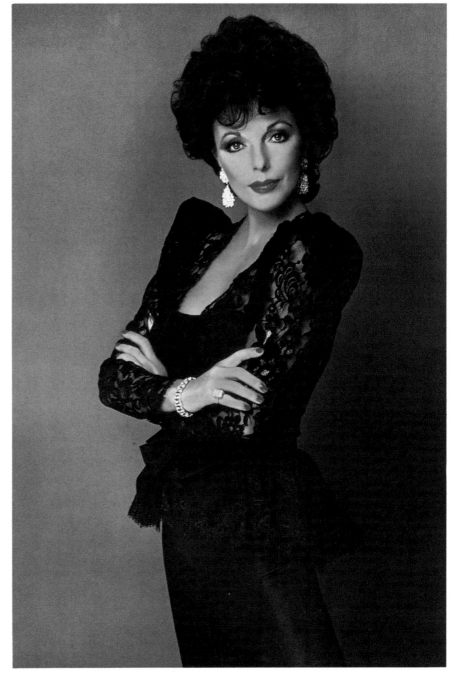

most of her time jetting between Europe and the States on various business ventures. She's had to develop a foolproof plan to ensure she arrives not only feeling relaxed but also looking good enough to face the cameras which follow her everywhere.

'I wear extremely comfortable clothes, either a tent dress or trousers, as loose as possible. And I always take a pair of boots one size

larger than usual to put on when I arrive.

'As soon as we take off, I remove my make-up and shoes, slather my face with moisturizer and drink lots of water. I have a bit of food and a couple of glasses of wine, put on my eye mask – a must for long-distance flights – and go to sleep.

'Then I wake up 15 minutes before we land and put my make-up on again – oh, and perfume, of course.'

# Mary Decker-Slaney

Her legs rate pin-up status and when they power her round a running track, hair streaming in the wind, it's easy to see why Mary Decker-Slaney is America's athletics sweetheart. When she's in running form Mary is an incredibly slender size 4 American (size 6 British). 'But I don't starve myself,' she says. 'In fact, I eat to put on weight. The only time I do anything in the line of "starvation" is before a race when I don't eat for anything up to six hours before – just drink loads of mineral water. I wouldn't recommend this build-up for anyone else – it just works for me.'

## Hair and skin

Despite her glamorous looks, she admits to a problem many women have. 'I have very fine permed hair and have to wash it frequently. I use a mild shampoo and Redken conditioner to keep it manageable.' Training in all weathers, she keeps her skin in good condition with Swiss La Prairie products, especially the moisturizer. To protect her lips from heat or cold, Mary uses Blisteze – a chapstick with a vaseline base.

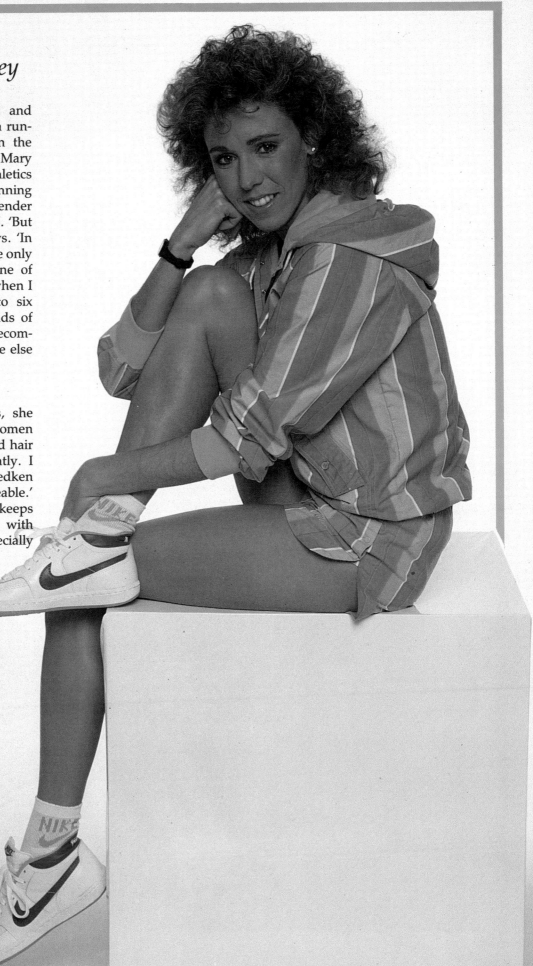

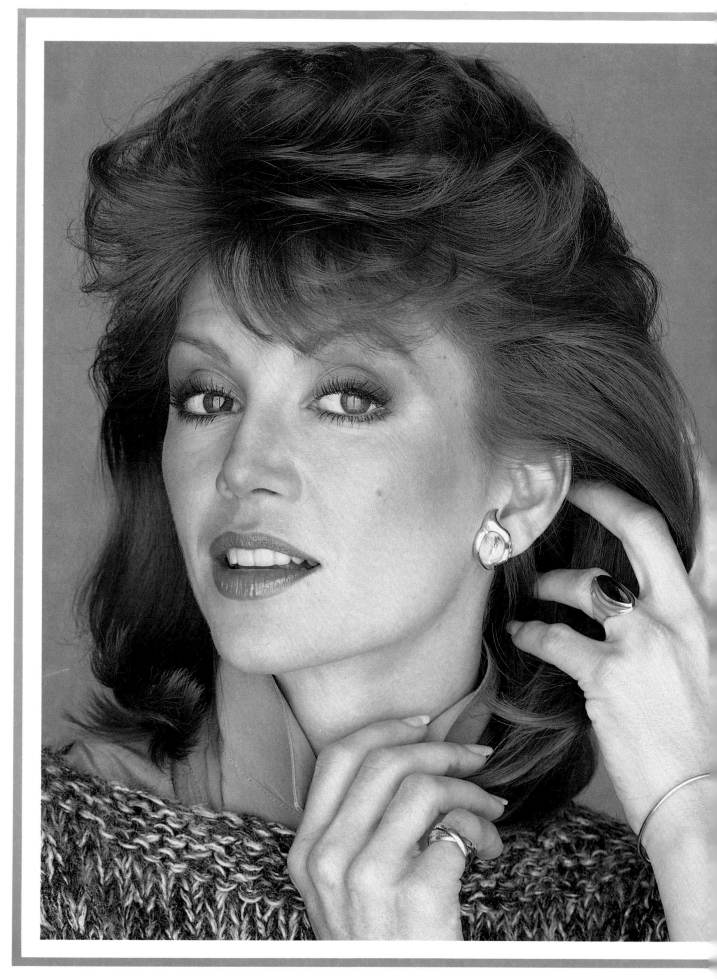

# Victoria Principal

Actress Victoria Principal's role as Pam Ewing in *Dallas* involves an early morning start – usually between 4 and 4.30 a.m. Nevertheless she has wonderfully wide-awake eyes. Her secret is 'enough sleep – my bed-down hour is almost always between 9 p.m. and 11 p.m. And in the morning, I use slices of cucumber or a cold compress laid across the lids for a few seconds shortly after I get up. During the day, if I'm tired, I try to take a short nap, whatever time it is. But I often find a short work-out or any form of exercise – which releases anti-depressant hormones into the bloodstream – is the best way to throw off that tired feeling.'

Victoria has written two books about her regimes: *The Body Principal* and *The Beauty Principal*.

## Sound advice

Her advice is sensible. 'I'd advise any woman to take advantage of every beauty article she can lay her hands on; glean advice from the skin care and cosmetics consultants in department stores; and talk to anyone who seems to know and care about cosmetics. However limited your funds, you can always find something to make you look and feel better.'

When she's not working, Victoria uses the minimum of make-up. 'Just moisturizer and blusher. If I'm in the sun I always wear a sun block cream and a visor. I find it very important to wear a creamy, moisturizing mascara. Waterproof mascara is drying, not good for lashes. Use it only when the situation warrants it – like when you're on holiday and swimming a lot.' She feels that good teeth are a big beauty asset. 'I go for dental check-ups more than is deemed necessary! And I always carry a vitamin E stick around with me to keep my lips moisturized.'

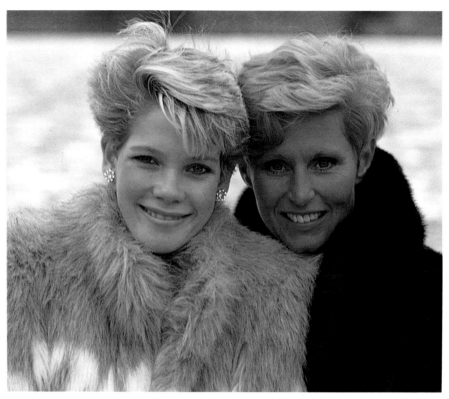

# Joanne Conway

When she was just 14 – an age when most young teenagers are just wondering vaguely what the future holds – Joanne Conway became the British ice-skating champion. And her looks are as dazzling as her skill on ice, although she says she does have problems.

'If I put on even 2 or 3 lb/about 1 kg, it shows around my middle – which doesn't look good when I'm performing. So I really have to be strict with myself. I eat three good meals a day – I need them for energy – but I have to cut out sweets, which I love, and junk food. I try to avoid canned drinks but I allow myself the odd diet cola. I usually practise five hours a day but even so, I need to do sit-ups and stretching exercises every night to make sure I stay really trim.'

Joanne's home is in North-east England but she spends most of her time in Colorado Springs, USA where she's coached by Carlo and Christa Fassi (with whom she is photographed above) who also trained John Curry and Robin Cousins.

## Hair and beauty

'I have my hair cut every four weeks or so in Colorado Springs – I keep it really short because that's what works best for competitions.' She has it highlighted every two months or so. 'I wash it every morning and blow-dry it with my head down – taking the brush from the nape of the neck towards the crown. Then I flick my head back and it all falls into place!'

Like any teenager, she loves experimenting with make-up but off the rink she keeps to a fairly light look – just moisturizer, a dark blue pencil to emphasize her eyes, mascara and lipgloss. Her feet are her fortune so she has regular chiropody treatments. 'I did develop athlete's foot at one stage from the heavy tights and boots but someone told me about Boots Cream E.45. It's magic – I also use it as a night cream because I've got dry skin and skating in cold conditions can aggravate it.'

## Paulene and Domino Stone

Paulene Stone has been an international cover girl since she won a *Woman's Own* model competition in 1958, when she was just 16. She has three children: Sophie, Domino and Harry, and lives in California. Domino looks uncannily like her father, actor Laurence Harvey, who died when she was five. But seeing them from behind, she and her mother could be sisters. Both are tall and slim with long, graceful necks and the same haircut.

### Living in the sun

Paulene's trademark used to be her long, luxuriant red hair 'but living in California and swimming every day, it made sense to have short hair. Mind you, I didn't do it with one drastic cut. I have the front lightened because, in strong sunlight, red hair can look garish.'

Her figure is still model-girl slim. 'I feel happiest at 9 st/57 kg – once I get up to 9½ st/60 kg I take action. I do yoga when I'm feeling flabby and in two weeks I can really change my shape. It's easier to keep weight off in California where we eat lots of fresh fruit, vegetables, jacket potatoes, brown bread and low-fat spreads. I'll have a beer with lunch, or wine with dinner and love to party occasionally. Living in the sun means being very careful about my skin and I never go out without Clinique's No. 19 sun block. Luckily the girls are beginning to learn how important sun blocks are too.'

### Sophie and Domino

With such a beauty-minded mother, it would make sense for Sophie and Domino to bombard her for advice. Not a bit. 'Sophie had skin problems in her teens, but they were cured when a skin specialist said what I'd been telling her for years – drink lots of water, cleanse properly and eat plenty of fruit and veg.'

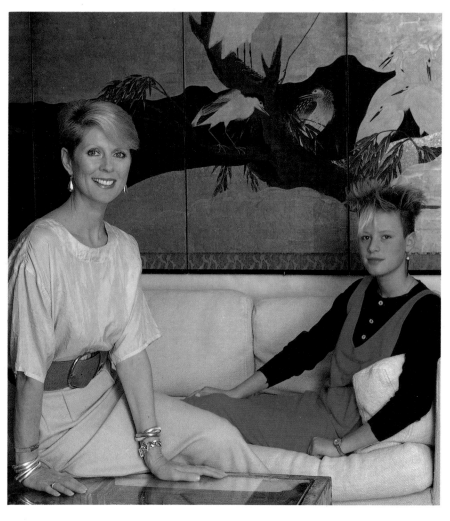

Domino, who has beautiful porcelain skin didn't ask Mum for tips either when she started wearing make-up. 'I just picked it up from Sophie. I use lipstick, blusher, mascara and eyeliner – but only a bit of everything. I wash my face with soap and water and I use a moisturizer. Now and again I give my skin a deep cleanse with a facial scrub. I wash my hair with whatever shampoo is lying around and I style it with gel.'

She won't let anyone but her mother's Los Angeles hairdresser cut her hair, but during term-time when she's at school in England she has it trimmed by a local barber.

### Beauty routine

Paulene's beauty routine is much more thorough. 'I wash my hair every day but find it gets too used to one shampoo so I vacillate between baby shampoo and Vidal Sassoon's or one by Leonard, plus conditioner. I use gel in the day or, if I'm going out at night, I backcomb the quiff and use lots of lacquer.

'I always use Boots' cleanser and toner but my moisturizer can vary from Boots to Lancôme to Dior. I use very little make-up – and what I do use is very lightly applied: Panstik as a base, applied with a damp sponge. A make-up artist persuaded me to try Panstik years ago and I've never found anything better. I love lots of rouge for a healthy look. I have lipsticks in all shades and I adore Chanel eye colours. Once I'm made-up I forget about my face. Two products that I've found invaluable for keeping make-up looking good all day are Elizabeth Arden's Eye Fix and Lip Fix.'

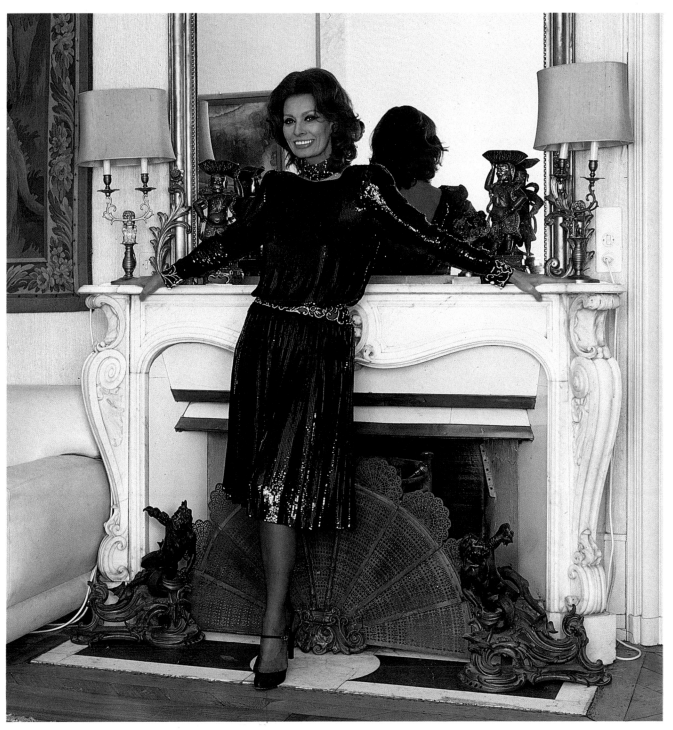

## Sophia Loren

'Journalists have often asked me, "What is your biggest beauty secret?" What can I say, I would wonder, struggling to find an answer that would be both honest and believable. I usually found a way to divert the conversation, but finally I have discovered that I do have a beauty secret. It is only a "secret" because you never hear or read about it, but I guarantee that it will make you more beautiful. It is a sense of inner peace. 'I can't take credit for it . . . it comes from my history, my experiences, my mother's strength, my personal faith, my children, so many things. And any tranquillity that I do have is fragile – but it is a great source of beauty. You can't sweat and strain yourself into being tranquil . . . it is more a matter of being receptive – to small pleasures in life and the satisfaction of goals achieved. You must be open to it. But there are some techniques to make you more receptive to tranquillity . . .'

133

**Organization.** Such a dull word! We like to pride ourselves on our spontaneity because somehow the freedom to be disorganized seems to belong to youth. But if you want to be tranquil and have a measure of peace in your life, you must be organized.

**Control.** I believe the greatest peace comes when we recognize the limits of our control. After you have done all you can, after you've bent every effort, you must recognize that you can't control everything. In some things you are not a director, but an actor. When you know this, you invite tranquillity.

**Goals.** Nothing brings more joy in life than a goal achieved. My children, my marriage, my career have all been the result of great struggle. I'm on familiar ground when I tell you that hard work and dedication to a goal have brought me greater happiness than anything else in my life. I hope that when I am 90, I will still be looking forward to working on some new project.

If your days are passing without any real sense of anticipation for what tomorrow holds, peace and tranquillity will elude you.

**Solitude.** I discovered early in life that I am my own best company, and I relish solitude as a means of regenerating myself, especially if I have problems or feel sad. Solitude that is chosen and not enforced is a true pleasure.

**Friendship.** I have only two or three close friends but they are so valuable to me. A true friend is a rare find. Such a person allows you to be truly yourself, for honesty is at the heart of friendship.

**Faith.** It is easy to lose touch with the spiritual side of one's nature and this is sad because it can be a great source of tranquillity and peace.'

# H.R.H. The Princess of Wales

*Woman's Own* have had the pleasure of the Princess of Wales's company on two occasions. In April 1984 she paid a private visit to the magazine and spent a morning touring the beauty, cookery, fashion and features departments – as well as art and production – to find out what makes a magazine tick.

She dazzled us all with her stunning eyes, beautiful skin and clever dress sense (she wore a severe Edwardian-style check coat with a soft white silk shirt and those now-famous seamed stockings with the cheeky bows) and her ability to cope with more than 100 new faces with charm and humour. The second occasion was when she presented our Children of Courage awards at Westminster Abbey in December 1985. As our picture shows, she was totally at ease with the young award-winners and made it a day they, and their proud parents, will never forget.

The Princess has described herself as 'scrawny' but to an observer's eye she is merely enviably slim. She keeps in shape by swimming as often as possible in the Buckingham Palace pool with Prince William and Prince Harry often joining in. She adores dance of any kind and tries to have two workouts a week.

When she first became engaged, Diana depended heavily on friends for fashion and make-up advice. (Her sister Jane used to work for *Vogue* magazine and it's no secret that Beauty Editor Felicity Clark was an enormous help.) Now, at 25, the Princess is an expert at knowing what suits her – both on the beauty and the fashion front. She loves browsing among the glossy cosmetic counters of Harvey Nichols in London's Knightsbridge – and has more than once shopped at the Lancôme counter. She likes their moisturizer – and their grey-blue eye pencil for framing those wonderful eyes. Like millions of other young women, she also appreciates the inexpensive natural products on sale in the Body Shop chain. The Princess feels good if her hair looks right. And, charged with the task of keeping her in tip-top shape is hairdresser, Richard Dalton of Headlines in London's South Kensington.

**Right:** The faces of courage in 1985 – the Princess of Wales congratulates the *Woman's Own* Children of Courage after a service at Westminster Abbey. **From bottom left (clockwise)** Steven Clarke, Darren Dunn, Joanne Baron, Jodie Woodward, with her mother Cheryl, Suhas Kulkarni, the Princess with Jamie Gavin, Samuel Heenan, Julie Malton, Sharon Allen and Sean Hedger.

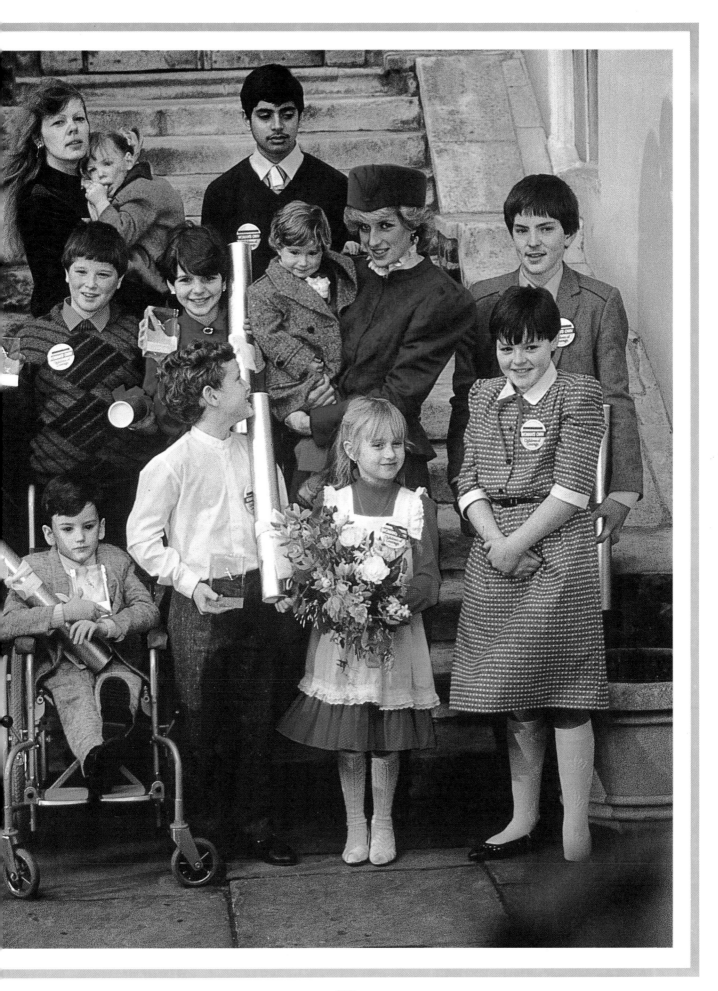

# Sunsense

*If you want to sport a glorious golden tan without damaging or drying out your skin, you have to protect and moisturize it. In less than 10 years, the burning urge to acquire a tan at any cost – using heavy oils to fry in or nothing at all – has turned to safety in 'numbers'. The numbered factors, first launched by Bergasol in 1977, flooded the market with protection ratios from 1 up to total sunblocks at 15 or more. The general guideline is that the higher the factor the better the screening, but all manufacturers give their own codes and formula explanations for different skin types.*

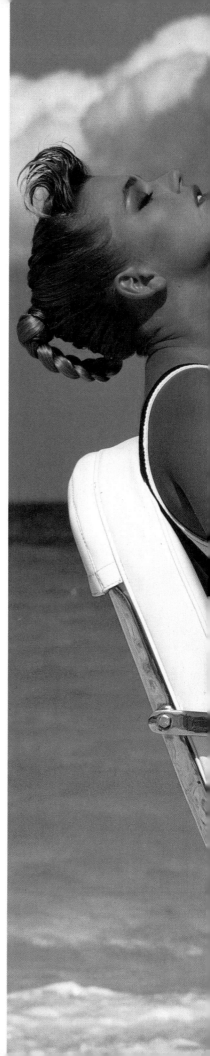

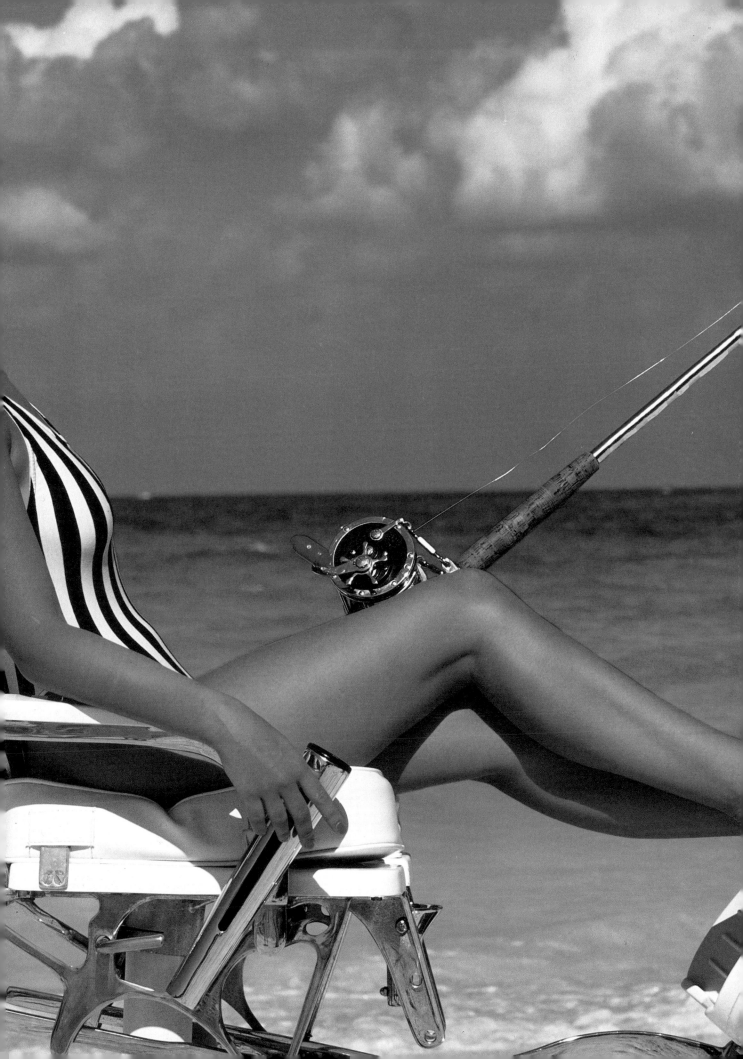

# Protection

This is the key factor when you seek the sun, and it comes in all forms – blocks, creams, mousses, gels and oils. And, we are now seeing cosmetic companies, as well as suntan product manufacturers, offering protective day moisturizers and foundations with SP (Sun Protection) factors. There are also creams to pre-condition your skin before baring all along with after-sun soothers and body moisturizers.

The sun's UV-B rays can quickly cause serious damage – reddening and burning of the skin – but dermatologists say it's also the longer UV-A rays which can cause permanent damage by ageing the skin prematurely. This has led to a turnabout in products and in particular sunbeds which are now designed to filter out both types of rays to a safer level of tanning.

Whether you intend to tan in or out of the sun, follow our survival plan to save your skin.

# Pre-sun precautions

It takes between three to four weeks for your skin to renew surface cells totally so before you dash out into the sun, give your body a top-to-toe once over. If you want to get an even tan, slough off dead surface cells for a smooth start (see Body Rub page 92).

How your skin tans is determined by three factors: age, genetic make-up and skin type (dry, normal or oily). Your skin will fall into one of four general groups:

**Very sensitive.** Red hair and freckles.

**Sensitive.** Light eyes, fair hair and peaches and cream skin.

**Average.** Probably mid-blue or brown eyes, mousy brown hair, some freckles.

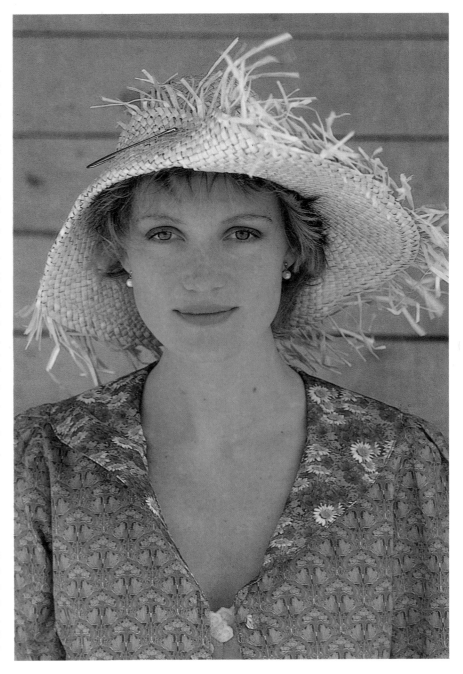

**Less sensitive.** Olive complexion, dark hair and eyes.

Whatever your skin type, you'll need a special sun block for the thinner, more susceptible skin under the eyes, backs of hands and knees, and neck and tops of feet. Generally, as you grow older your skin becomes thinner which makes it more sun-sensitive.

A tan is caused by the skin producing a brown substance called

*A sun hat is essential at any age to keep skin looking good by keeping off the sun's hazardous rays.*

melanin which rises to the surface and acts as a barrier against the sun's UV rays. Unfortunately, most skins need more protection than mother nature has given them to filter out the hazardous rays. It takes some time for the melanin to be activated and some of the painful burning and damage can be done in

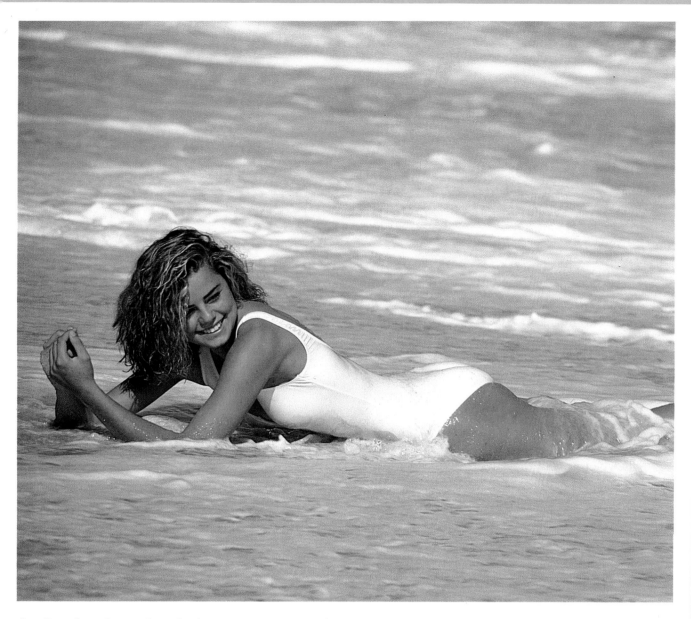

the first few days of sunbathing. The general rule when sunbathing is to do it gradually and not when the sun is at its peak around midday. It's always a good idea to give yourself some pre-tanning boosters.

**Sunbeds** are great for activating the melanin before you go out into the sun. Invest in a course of treatments before going on holiday and remember that your skin can still dry out, so always moisturize afterwards. When under any sunbed *always* wear goggles to protect your eyes.

**Pre-tan creams and lotions** Some recommend that you start a few days before going on holiday, some

are two-week treatments. They work by stimulating the skin's melanin.

## In the sun
You don't have to be on a beach to need a sunscreen; shopping, sight-seeing or walking to the beach can prove hazardous since UV rays can penetrate through hazy clouds or reflect from sand, water and white buildings. Protect your skin even if you are just wandering in and out of the shops.

When buying sun protection products take note of your skin type. Whether you use a cream, oil or lotion is a matter of preference but make sure the sun protection

*Enjoy the benefits of sea-bathing but always shower off afterwards to remove all traces of salt and re-apply sun protection cream. Alternatively use a water-resistant product.*

factor is suitable for the degree of sensitivity of your skin.

**Very sensitive skins** Always carry a sunblock for critical spots and always wear a high-protection cream. If your skin reacts violently to sunshine and turns extra dry, red, blotchy, itchy and swollen, then opt for one of the hypo-allergenic brands which are usually fragrance-free since perfume can trigger off allergies under the sun. And don't try for more than a gentle honey-coloured suntan.

**Sensitive skins** On days one to four, use a high-protection cream all over. On day five, switch to a cream or lotion with a sun protection factor of 4, 5 or 6.

**Less sensitive skins** On days one to two, use a medium-protection cream. On day three, switch to a low-protection cream or lotion if you can see your skin is coping.

**Average skins** On days one to two, use a medium-protection cream. On day three, switch to a low-protection oil to help to deepen that golden glow. If you're a water baby and tend to forget to re-apply your sun protection cream, then be sure to choose a waterproof or water-resistant product. These creams contain polymers which increase their staying power on the skin.

Remember, when dipping in and out of the sea or pool, that salt and chlorine have a drying effect on the skin – particularly the face. Take a can of Evian water facial spray and wash away salt and chlorine on the spot.

## After-sun soothers

At the end of the day always shower and rinse your hair well and seal in your tan by moisturizing well. After-sun products arc included in most suntan ranges – offering everything from soothing agents like *Aloe vera* and allantoin.

There's no reason why you shouldn't use your favourite body moisturizer or body milk after the sun since all you have to make sure of is that your skin doesn't dry out. Apply generously after a bath or shower.

Some after-sun products contain self-tanning ingredients, promising that your tan will gently improve overnight. If you have caught a slight sunburn, stay out of the sun and treat with calamine lotion.

## Fake tans

If you are loath to go out baring a lily-white body, some of the fake tan products can give a hint of a tan. Unfortunately, they don't always give an even colour since some parts of the skin (particularly the dry areas) will absorb more of the cream than others.

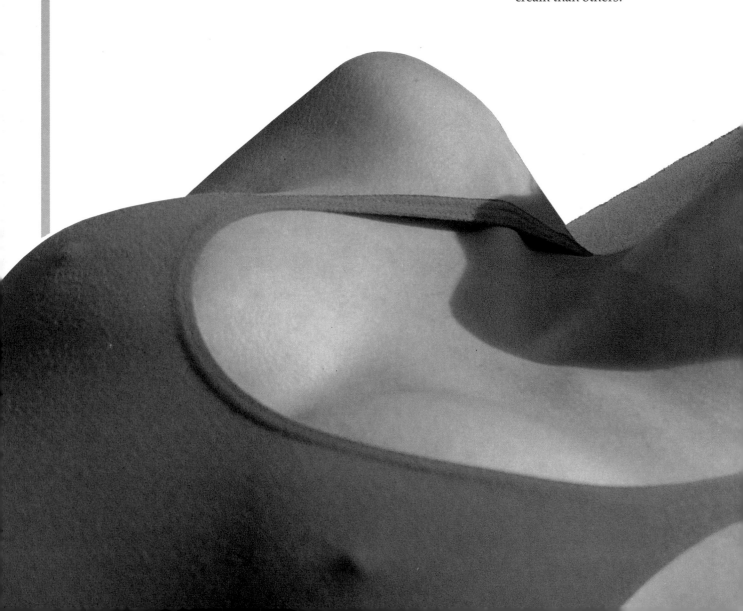

## Protect and feel comfortable

### Hair

Coloured, permed or tinted hair is vulnerable in the sun. The UV (ultra-violet) rays can soon fade a tint or frizz a perm. The best protection is a sunhat – of the wide-brimmed straw variety – or just a scarf to cover the head when the sun is at its peak around midday. If you scrunch your hair up in a covered elastic band, don't forget that those sensitive areas around the nape of the neck and shoulders will burn easily if left exposed. Protect with a high filter sun protection cream or gel.

Swimming is great for the body but if you're diving in and out of the sea or pool, remember to look after your hair. Always rinse away salt (which can strip away hair's natural oils if left to dry on hair) and chlorine under the shower and give hair an extra treatment conditioner.

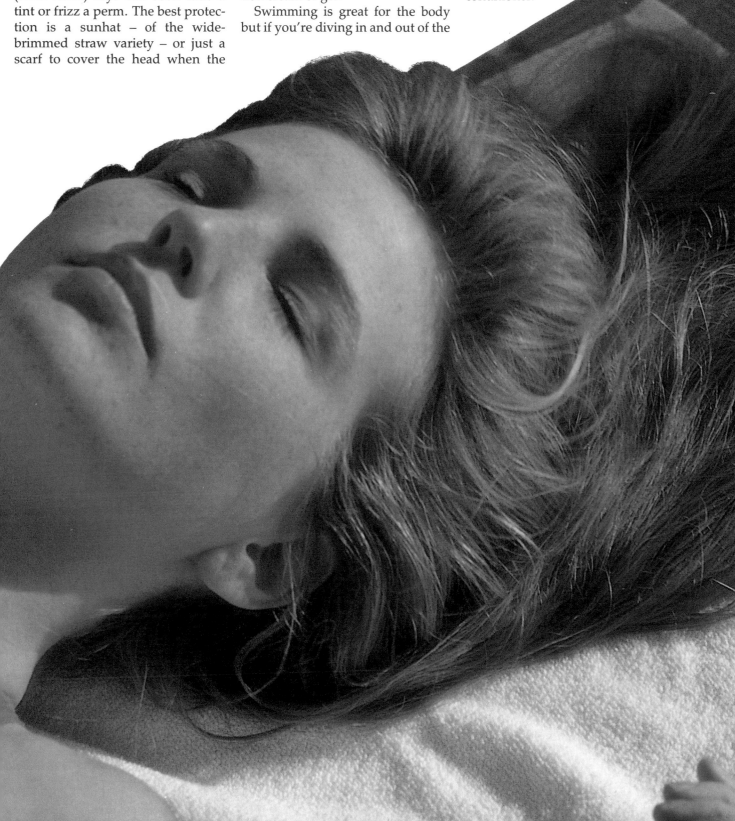

If you want to give hair a little more gloss while in the sun, slick on some of the new styling creme gels which can give a wet-look or simply add extra body. You can apply most of them on wet or dry hair.

Look out for the colour-reviving gels. These range from camomile for blonde hair to chestnut for dark hair and you just comb them through to revive either natural or tinted colour.

For particularly dry or damaged hair, opt for a gel which contains UV filters to block out the sun's harmful rays. They can be applied to wet or dry hair – simply comb through.

Although it's all right to have your hair coloured just before going on holiday, it's best to have it permed at least one month before, giving it a chance to settle down and regain some of its natural oils.

You're going to be exposing your hair to enough heat in the sun, so avoid overuse of high-speed hair-dryers and heated tongs and rollers. If you have to use rollers, wind a strip of sponge round them first to protect the hair and discourage tangles.

## Sunglasses

An attractive fashion accessory, sunglasses also provide invaluable protection for the eyes. Because lenses are easily scratched on the beach, choose a pair of sunglasses with good scratch-resistant properties and, if you are not used to wearing spectacles, opt for a pair with lighter plastic frames.

The three main types of lenses – gradient, reactolite and polarized – all absorb almost all harmful UV rays. If you wear glasses anyway, you may prefer reactolite lenses which darken at the first glimmer of sunshine. Otherwise, opt for clip-ons to fit your ordinary glasses.

Remember that even when you're in the shade, UV light can reflect from surrounding white buildings, so keep your glasses on.

## Clothes

Choose pale colours for your holiday wardrobe; not only because they look fresh and cool, but because white reflects away the sun's rays which tend to be absorbed by darker colours.

If you want to avoid prickly-heat or excess perspiration, make sure your cover-ups are made of natural fibres which absorb sweat easily and don't aggravate the skin. Cottons are cooler. Polyester and nylon mixes trap the heat and prevent the skin from breathing.

With cut-away swimsuits, you may find your skin tingling in those sensitive lower back and upper thigh areas. Always carry a T-shirt to the beach to protect your back and shoulders if they start to tingle. Another holiday essential is a kanga lightweight wrap-around to cover knees and tops of shins when you're sitting outside for lunch even if you think you're in the shade.

Look out for the summer ranges of underwear in 100 per cent cotton. And, if you don't want to wear tights or stockings, make sure legs are hair-free (see page 147) and give them an extra sheen with a rich moisturizing body lotion or oil.

Protect feet on the beach from sharp pebbles or burning sands with a pair of cheap and cheerful jolly jellies – pumps or slingbacks – available from most chain stores.

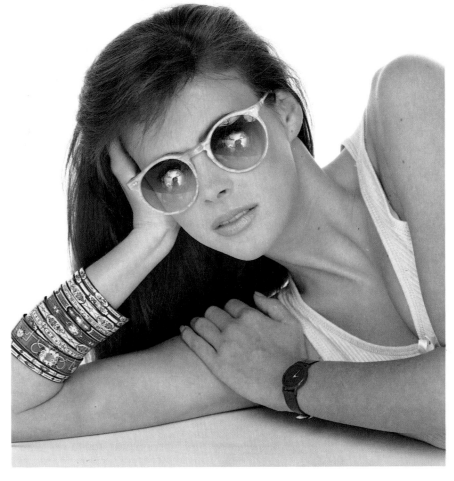

*Never go into the sun without a pair of glasses and (right) some kind of cover-up for sensitive shoulders.*

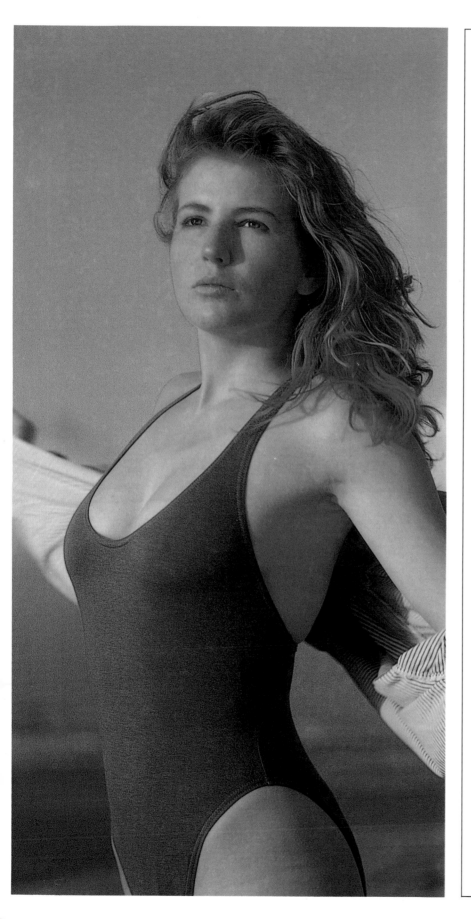

## Seven ways to exploit your tan

**1** Some people think that exfoliation scrubs off a tan, but this is totally untrue. On the contrary, whisking off the tiny flakes instantly livens up a tan and helps it to last longer.

**2** Once the skin is scrupulously clean and smooth, give it some extra special night care with a touch of oil. Oils penetrate more rapidly than creams because they filter through the hair follicle not just through the horny layers of surface cells.

**3** If you want to go bare-faced and show off clear, golden skin, you can. There's no need to cover up with foundation. Tinted moisturizers help to even out skin tones and to make you look barefaced when you're not.

**4** Enhance your eyes by keeping them clear and sparkling with an eyewash or eyedrops. Frame them with lashes enhanced with a coating of mascara. Shimmer the lids with sandy gold and summery bronze shadows.

**5** For a healthy glow, emphasize cheekbones with a dusting of golden-flecked blusher.

**6** A trick for lips is to protect them with a lipsalve or sunscreen. When the sun goes down, slick on a glossy lip tint or lip gloss.

**7** Extend the powers of your beauty bag with one box of tricks – Ultra Glow Powder. This golden-flecked powder can be used on the face as shader, contourer, highlighter or blusher. You can use it wet as an eyeliner or to liven up your eye shadows. You can even add a dusting to your favourite body lotion to give your skin an extra sheen.

# Finishing Touches

*Being well groomed isn't just being fashionably 'together'. If your slip's showing or there's a ladder in your tights you can spoil a chic look – even if you've pressed those pleats in your tailored skirt. Take an overall look at yourself and see if you pass the grooming test.*

*First, your hair. Does it look well cut and shiny? Second, your make-up. Does it blend in with your clothes in complementary colour schemes?*

*Finishing touches don't stop at that extra dusting of powder to prevent shine, or dash of lipline to prevent lipstick creasing – they extend to teeth, hands and feet. Take a look at one of your most expressive assets – your smile. When was the last time you had your teeth professionally cleaned by a hygienist? Take a look at your hands.*

*Are they 'dishpan' rough or soft to touch? Are your nails nicely shaped or chipped? A regular manicure is essential not only for healthy nails but, under the well groomed tag, for perfect polish. If you want to feel light-footed, give yourself a regular pedicure and see a registered chiropodist for professional toenail trimming and hard skin removal.*

*Baring your body can be more than revealing. Are you as hair-free and smooth as you would like? On the following pages we show you how to look well groomed both in and out of clothes.*

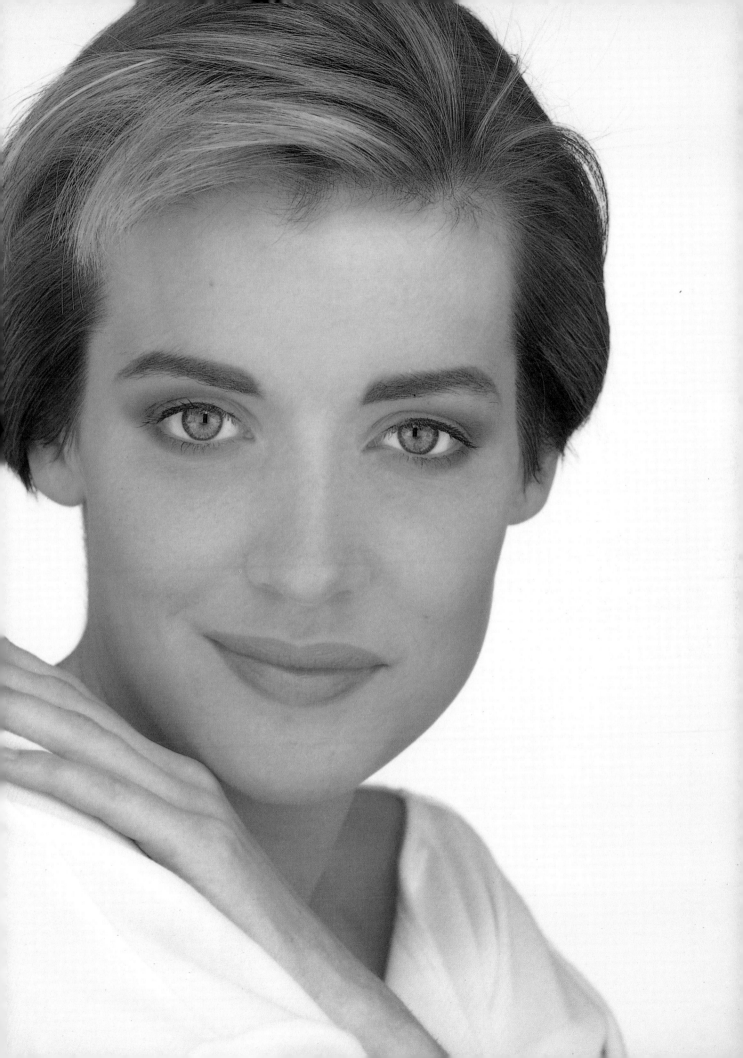

## Styled for success

Sophia Loren says that her favourite 'uniform' is a long black mac, and a pair of well-cut black trousers worn with a silk shirt topped with 'a really beautiful long scarf'. 'In this I can go almost anywhere', she says. The art of dressing beautifully, she proves, is not how much you spend but the way you put a 'look' together. Here's how you too can look terrific.

**Be colour conscious.** Pick a basic colour theme – and stick to it. Decide whether you look best in black, navy, beige or grey and buy major items such as suits, coats, jackets and pants in these colours. You can always add bright touches with boldly coloured shirts, sweaters and scarves. Match shoes, boots and bags accordingly. It's better to have four items that mix and match than seven or eight garments that look terrific on their own but team with nothing else.

**Be selective.** Go through your wardrobe and take out anything that doesn't work for its living – the impulse buys, the slightly too tight skirts, the fashion item that faded fast! Make a list of what's lacking to pull a look together and buy carefully over the next year.

**Be extravagant.** Instead of two or three impulse buys, promise yourself one luxury item – it could be a designer scarf, a cashmere sweater, a Liberty print shawl, a silk shirt or a

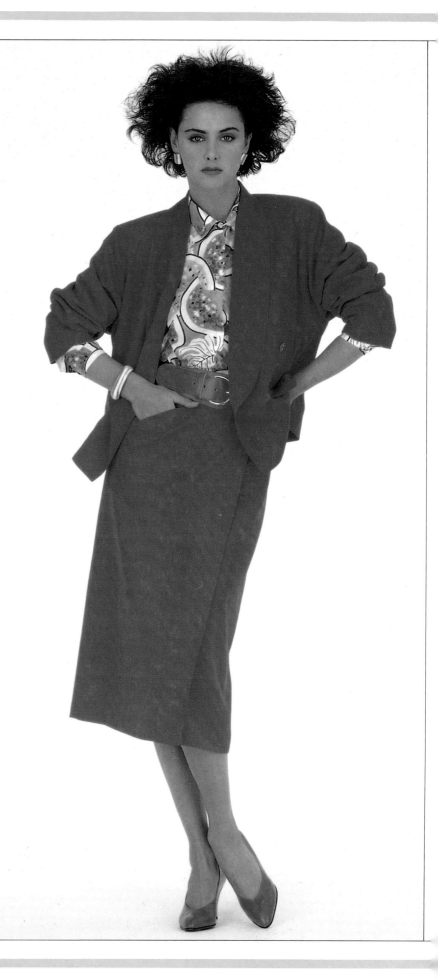

leather jacket – anything that will add an extra dash of excitement to your everyday clothes. It pays to go for investment dressing now and again – quality items will last for years.

**Be clever.** You can wear the same quality outfits year in, year out if you watch fashion trends without following them slavishly. Always adjust hemlines fractionally to fit in with the current style, look out for the little touches that are 'in' – the ways to tie a scarf, the latest shade of tights, the newest inexpensive bangles. Study fashion pages in magazines and fashion counters of department stores for the budget looks.

**Be you.** With a complete outfit already put together for them, women still want their clothes to be individual. Whether you're on a limited budget or can afford a charge account there are ways to look stylish while retaining your individuality. Most towns nowadays have nearly new shops – great hunting grounds for classy clothes at cut-down prices.

Try antique markets for pieces of lace or Victorian jewellery that will add a distinctive note to a plain shirt, for instance. Or build up a versatile collection of belts and jewellery that will turn a plain black dress into something that bears your own distinctive style.

# Hair removal

There are various ways of removing excess hair. Some you can do yourself but for a more permanent solution you should seek professional treatment.

### Waxing
Undoubtedly the most effective and lasting method of warding off unwanted hair from areas like legs and bikini line is waxing although, of course, the hair will regrow in three to six weeks. Traditionally, it is done with runny, melted wax applied to the skin with a spatula. Seconds later a fabric strip is applied on top of the wax, then quickly pulled away from the skin, taking the unwanted hair with it.

This method is highly recommended, providing the hairs are removed from their follicles. But it needs care – and nerve! You can do it at home but it is best done professionally.

Bikini-line hair removal in particular is best left to the professionals. This part of the body is more sensitive that the legs because it contains larger veins and lymph glands. Shaving often causes a reaction here – possibly a rash, infected follicles or ingrown hairs.

Vera Jovic, beauty therapist at Glemby in Harvey Nichols, London, describes how bikini-line waxing is done professionally: 'We clean the skin with surgical spirit and dust powder over it so the wax clings to the hair, not to the skin. Wax hardens in seconds and only a skilled beautician knows the point at which to pull it away before this happens.'

Some beauticians use cool wax, a method which is suitable for fine hair, but less effective on the stronger leg and bikini-line hair. Used on this stronger growth, the hair may be just broken off rather than removed from the roots.

Cold wax strips are ideal for use at home: you simply press the impregnated strips on to the skin and immediately whisk them off.

Deal with the regrowth on holiday with tweezers, which, like wax, take the hair from the follicle. Obviously this is not practical for general use but is an effective temporary measure.

### Shaving
If you still prefer to shave, do it carefully with a disposable razor or an electric razor that cannot nick the skin. Shaving dries the skin, so be sure to apply a moisturizer afterwards.

### Depilatories
If you just want to get rid of fine leg hair, mousse hair remover is effective. Simply squirt the mousse on, spread it over the legs, leave for eight minutes, then rinse off. It's fast-acting and works, we found, even on quite strong hair. Depilatories are effective for underarm hair too, as waxing requires a certain amount of regrowth before you can repeat the treatment.

Hair remover also comes in a roll-on form, for easy application, but it is essential to do a patch test first with any depilatory because sensitive skin may suffer a reaction.

### Electrolysis
Electrolysis is the permanent solution to unwanted facial hair, hair around the nipples and the 'zip line' which is the trickle of hair that can grow from the tummy to the top of the bikini line. (For hair around nipples and the odd facial hair, tweezing is the only other method of removal which may be used. Never try to wax or shave facial hair at home.)

Don't be afraid of electrolysis; it's a simple and painless treatment, whereby a small electric current deadens the papilla which feeds the hair root. After only a few treatments your skin will be free of hair for ever.

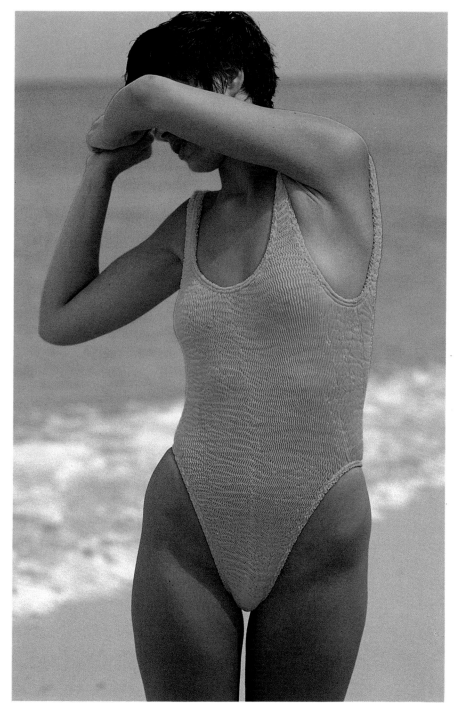

## Manicure

The fashion for nail shapes has changed over the years. But it's best to keep to the natural look with nail tips short and slightly oval – not long and pointed.

**1** *Using an emery board, file nails in one stroke from side to centre of nail.*

**2** *Soak nails in warm, soapy water for a couple of minutes to soften cuticles and to wash away any traces of oily nail polish remover. Softened cuticles are easier to push back and any hangnails are easier to trim.*

**3** *If your creamy cuticle remover doesn't come with a brush, apply it with an orange stick covered with cotton wool. Using the hoof edge of the stick, push back cuticles and, with pointed edge, clean underneath nails. Wash away remover.*

**4** *Always use proper manicure clippers or scissors which are designed specifically for the job. Only hangnails and excess skin should be neatly trimmed. Never cut into the cuticle or you may find it will harden and crack.*

**5** *Nails that split easily, chip, flake or simply snap off need extra care. If you're not going to wear nail polish for a few hours, then condition nails by applying a nail-care cream to the entire area, massaging it well into the cuticle. Then use a buffing cream and chamois leather polisher.*

**6** *For perfectly polished nails, first apply a clear base coat to stop nails discolouring. Paint nails in three strokes – centre and then each side. Next add two coats of polish. Finish with a clear top coat for extra protection. Make sure each coat is allowed to dry between applications.*

### Bleaching

Finally, for hair best left where it is, there's bleach. Great for facial hair and dark hair on arms, the treatment is available in beauty salons, or can be done with one of the many home bleach kits. Bleaching can last successfully for up to two months.

To make your own bleaching solution, mix 20 volume peroxide (available from a chemist) with an

*Waxing, depilatories or electrolysis are ways to deal with unwanted body hair but bleaching is an answer too. Always remember to patch-test first.*

equal part of water. Apply to hair with cotton wool. Leave for 10 to 12 minutes and rinse off with warm water.

As with depilatories, always patch-test bleach first to check there's no adverse skin reaction, and apply moisturizer after use.

REMEMBER: Beautiful hands don't stop at the nails. Always pamper your skin with a moisturizing hand-cream. Try to cut down on some of the wear and tear you give your hands around the house. Always wear rubber gloves for washing up, cotton gloves for housework and gardening gloves when weeding. Carry an emery board in your bag, so you can do an emergency manicure before a break gets too bad.

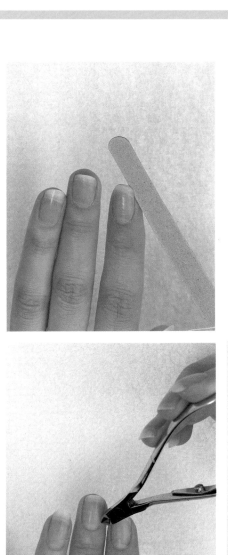

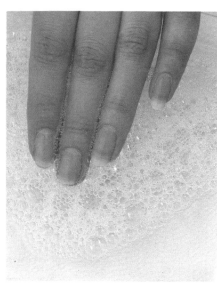

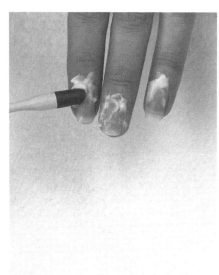

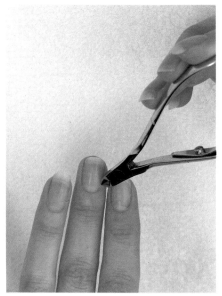

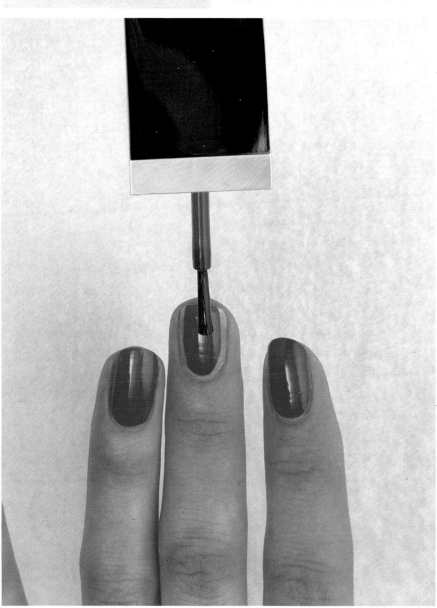

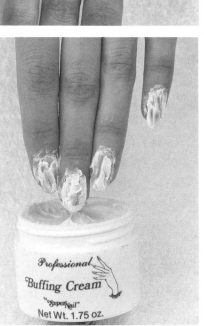

## On your toes

Healthy feet put a smile on your face: if they're 'killing' you, it shows. It's been estimated that before reaching the age of 20, about 70 per cent of us have developed foot ailments of some kind. One pair of badly fitting shoes in childhood can be enough to trigger off painful growth and later foot problems.

With today's emphasis on active sports, keep-fit, dancing and jogging, feet come in for a fair share of battering so they need extra care and attention. Here are a few pointers on how to keep your feet in trim.

### Massage

Massage tired feet with your own pampering treatment. Place a small towel on one thigh, and bring the foot of the opposite leg up to rest on the towel. Now massage hand or foot lotion into the foot, working from base of toes up to the ankle, pressing firmly with the pad of your thumb along the sole. Massage each toe individually, moving from base

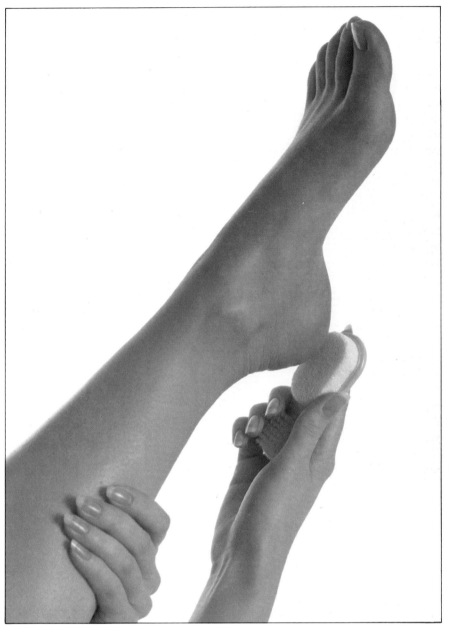

to top and pulling each one very gently.

When your feet are smooth, fragrant and flexible, it's time to pedicure and polish.

### Nail tips

1 Using specially rounded clippers like those in the Scholl range, clip nails straight across and not too short, so they are just a fraction longer than the tip of the toe.
2 Clean nails with an orange stick and gently push back cuticles – never try to cut off hangnails or pierce the skin with pointed scissors. If you have to remove hard

*Unhappy feet reflect in your face so give them regular care and ensure shoes fit correctly.*

cuticle skin, soften first with cuticle cream and then use a liquid remover.
3 Try using toe spacers (foam wedges or cotton wool balls to separate toes) so that you don't smudge the nail varnish.
4 Give nails a base coat to protect them from varnish stains and provide a smooth base for your nail varnish. Apply two coats and finally add a top coat to guard against unattractive chipping.

## Foot problems

Most of us were born with perfectly structured feet – 26 bones arranged to form a series of arches; a framework supported by ligaments, muscles and tendons through which runs a network of arteries, veins and nerves. All this gives us the flexibility to walk, run, jump, stand on tiptoe or simply stand.

Pressure on the nerves of your feet caused by even the most minor foot ailments, can give you backache and pains in other parts of your body.

**Corns** are the result of friction and shoe pressure on the skin of the feet when the skin is squashed between the bone and the shoe. Corns do not have roots and may be due to a structural deformity but the most common cause is badly fitting shoes which give continuous irritation. Avoid chemical cures for corns but you can use pads to alleviate them. If they persist, have them professionally treated by a state registered chiropodist.

**Callouses** are also caused by friction and the build up of hard dead skin. Unlike corns, which are usually on the tops or tips of toes, callouses can grow over any bony prominence, like the balls of feet. If pressure on the nerves causes a burning sensation, use specially formulated pads to soften and protect. You can stop build-up with a pumice stone, but never attempt to cut callouses yourself – always have them treated by a state registered chiropodist.

**Verrucae** are often mistaken for corns but they are contagious, painful and can spread if left untreated. Foot warts caused by a virus, verrucae usually appear on the soles of the feet. Children running about barefoot in the school gymn or swimming pool area pick them up easily. Make sure that during medical treatment infected feet are covered, own towels are used, and that cork or bath mats are not shared with anyone else.

**Bunions** are caused by a thickening of the skin at the head of a metatarsal bone forming a painful, obtrusive lump at the side of the foot. Shoes that are ill-fitting or pointed, or stockings that are too short, can often cause bunions. You can alleviate the pain with soothing lotions and pad the bunions with foam shields but if you want to get rid of them, see a specialist for treatment.

**Chilblains** are caused by bad circulation and cold weather. Symptoms are redness, tingling and an itching sensation which results in a painful swelling, usually around the heel area. Shoes can aggravate; apply ointments to soothe, do regular foot exercises and take hot and cold foot bath dips to stimulate the blood supply.

**Athlete's foot** is a skin disease caused by a fungus, and not strictly confined to athletes! This fungus thrives in warm, damp conditions and, like verrucae, is highly contagious. Symptoms are itchy rashes, split skin between toes, and blisters. Treat with a specially formulated athlete's foot liquid or powder. Change socks or tights daily and don't spread it around on the bathroom mat – stand on your own towel!

**Excessive perspiration** is an embarrassing problem – not the wetness but the accompanying odour. Caused by a disorder of the sweat glands, it can be relieved effectively by using special foot powder containing both anti-perspirant and deodorant ingredients. Daily washing and frequent changing of footware are essential.

**Ingrowing toenails** are generally caused by improper trimming – cutting the nails down at the sides instead of straight across – but heredity, injury and infection can all be contributory factors. The nail grows into the flesh, causing considerable pain. Professional treatment should be sought as soon as possible as it can be difficult to remedy if left too late.

---

### Foot tips

● Try to vary your shoe heel heights. Wearing high heels all day and all evening not only makes the feet swell but throws out the spine and is bad for posture.

● Wear well fitting shoes that don't pinch and squeeze.

● Give your feet a break by walking around barefoot at home or wearing exercise sandals.

Fit foot-flexing exercises into your day:

● Stand on tiptoes, hold, then replace heels on floor.

● Stand on a thick book and curl your toes over the edge.

● Flex and extend your foot so toes move first towards you then point away, like a ballet movement.

● Draw up your toes to increase foot arch.

● Spread your toes often if they're cramped after years of wearing pinch-toed shoes.

● To prevent the formation of tough, hard skin and callouses, feet should be given daily abrasive treatment in the bath with a pumice stone and/or loofah. Once a week you could also give them a sloughing treatment: rub a mixture of vegetable oil and coarse sea salt into the feet before getting into the bath.

# Teeth

There's nothing more dazzlingly attractive than a good set of teeth. But if you want every tooth to be a pearl you must put your money where your mouth is – like the Americans, who consider cosmetic dentistry as vital as any facelift.

The dentist, once thought of as the next best thing to a torturer in horror films, is becoming more akin to a beauty therapist. The modern dental surgery is a place to indulge yourself. You can go there to relax, in comfort, while you have your looks transformed, then walk away with a smile you know you can wear proudly. Now there are exciting new alternatives to the traditional silver fillings and bridges, crowns and stiff faces, deep fillings and gas. While dentists' surgeries have been changing, so too have our mouths. Fifty per cent of five-year-olds in Britain are now completely decay-free; that's more than ever before. But there's no need for us to be complacent; new problems arise as soon as we solve the old ones. What's more, a quarter of Britons over 25 have none of their natural teeth left. This is largely because of gum disease, where bacteria and germs build up on teeth and form a film called plaque, which causes serious damage to gums and teeth. A worrying nine in 10 of us have some gum disease, which is characterized by bleeding or swollen red gums (healthy gums are pale pink and firm). But the good news is that with good habits – careful thorough cleansing with the right tools, regular check-ups and healthy eating – tooth decay and gum disease are preventable.

## Improving your smile
Once your dental health is under control, you'll probably become more concerned with how your teeth look, for researchers have discovered that the two go hand in hand. Here are details of the cosmetic dental techniques currently available.

**Light-cured veneers** can be used instead of crowns to hide stains or close gaps between teeth. A thin plastic cover is moulded into place and then hardened in 30 seconds with a harmless, bright blue light beam. Compared with crowns, they minimize the necessity for drilling and anaesthetics, so lessen pain and time.

**Dentine bonding,** a quick, painless alternative to deep fillings, fills the gaps at the tops of teeth caused by shrinking gums and toothbrush wear. The exposed yellow root is simply covered with a bonding material, thus avoiding the drilling of good teeth.

**Maryland and Rochette bridges** can solve the problem of one of two missing teeth. The old solution was a small plastic or metal denture or, alternatively, drilling away what might be good teeth on either side of the gap to make an ordinary bridge.

The new bridges (some of which were developed from space technology at the NASA space laboratories in Florida) do away with the drilling of good teeth and wearing plates.

A Rochette bridge is attached by tiny metal wings, invisible when smiling or talking, which are bonded to the back of the good teeth on either side with resin. The Maryland bridge has a fine metal strand instead of wings and is fixed in the same way. The Rochette is cheaper, quicker and less painful than the old-style bridges.

**White fillings** in back teeth have banished that silver laugh which reveals your dental history. These fillings look good, and are tougher now than the originals, which came into use in the 1960s and could only be used in front teeth. But they have not yet stood the test of time.

**News for migraine sufferers** is that dentists who specialize in occlusal problems (the way our teeth bite together) have cured some migraine sufferers by analyzing and modifying their bite.

## Comfort factors
Many of us fear a visit to the dentist because of the discomfort that results but, here too, modern techniques are improving the patients' lot.

**Relative analgesia** (RA) is a new alternative to general anaesthetic and intravenous sedation for the nervous patient. You put on a nose-piece, which brings oxygen and nitrous oxide to make you feel half asleep but still with-it enough to speak and hear.

It has no smell, requires no starving or special preparation and has none of the risks of an anaesthetic. It relaxes you and helps to reduce pain.

**Single-tooth injections** will deaden some teeth without giving you a stiff face and numb tongue for hours afterwards.

## Tooth protectors
Treatments that can protect your teeth are assuming much greater importance.

**Fissure sealant** is a plastic material which can be applied, in liquid form, to the biting surfaces of back teeth as they come through in the mouth, usually when children reach the age of seven or eight. The plastic sets hard and helps to prevent the teeth from decay.

**Jet cleaners** remove plaque and stains quickly, effectively and with little discomfort, but hand scaling still produces the best results.

**Facts on fluoride** Fluoride is a substance that occurs naturally in rocks and some water sources. Harmless at the right concentration levels, fluoride is added to drinking

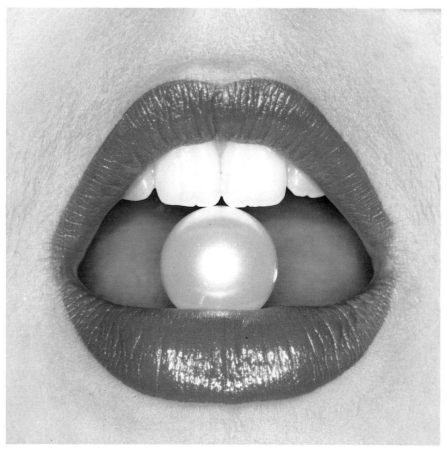

*New developments in dentistry mean that everyone can have teeth like pearls!*

water in parts of Britain because it has been shown beyond doubt to be very effective in strengthening teeth against decay. It is also added to most toothpastes. Fluoride toothpastes promote remineralisation and can prevent very tiny cavities in teeth from enlarging, so that they don't need fillings.

If the level of fluorides in your local water supply is low, it might be worth giving fluoride tablets to children aged between two and 12. Dosage should be geared to water supply concentration.

## Tooth problems

Wear, and particularly, stained teeth and bad breath can be a worry and effect your self-confidence.

**Tooth wear** becomes an important new problem as we are now keeping our natural teeth longer. Over the years the way we bite can wear down enamel and dentine and this can be speeded up if a faulty crown or bridge has been fitted. Obsessive brushing can mean you are literally brushing away your teeth, especially after they have been softened by the acids in food and drink.

**Tooth staining** is caused mainly by nicotine, coffee, tea, red wine and betel-nut chewing (popular among Asians). If your teeth are stained, cut down on these and have professional polishes done more often. Smokers should avoid abrasive toothpowders – they wear away the teeth. More serious staining which cannot be removed easily requires a veneer treatment.

**Bad breath** (halitosis) is rarely caused by tooth decay, but commonly caused by gum disease. If you're dentally fit, there may be an underlying cause, so seek medical advice. Mouthwashes (except those prescribed by your doctor or dentist) and mouth sprays are largely cosmetic and their effects often short-lived.

## Brushing up on prevention

● Have a dental check-up every six months; at home, look after your own teeth and brush those of any children under eight years.

● Choose toothbrushes which have a small head, nylon filaments with rounded tips, and perhaps an angled handle for improved manoeuvring.

● Toothpaste with fluoride is best (more than 90 per cent contain fluoride). Squeeze $\frac{1}{2}$in/ 1cm of toothpaste on the brush.

● Brushing techniques differ, but your hygienist can show you the best way for you. Try to cover all tooth surfaces, especially around the gums, with gentle circular or vibratory movements. Brush for three minutes, twice a day (morning and night). Even better, keep a travelling toothbrush in your bag and brush after lunch, too.

● Floss is vital for cleaning between the teeth. Slide the fine thread between your teeth and scrape off the plaque, ideally every day.

● Wooden dental sticks are a good alternative to floss. So is floss tape. Check occasionally on how thoroughly you've been cleaning with a plaque-disclosing tablet.

● A healthy diet for teeth is one which is low in sugary foods and drinks. A lot of foods have a hidden sugar content – even savoury foods, like baked beans and canned soup. If you must have something sugary, eat it with, rather than between, your meals. Never drink or snack at night after brushing.

# Beauty at any Stage

*As we grow older – indeed, soon after we've physically grown up – our bodies begin to run down. Circulation and cell renewal are not so speedy, sebaceous glands which provide oil to condition and lubricate the skin and give it a thin, protective layer to seal in vital moisture, cease to function so profusely. The connective tissue in the skin's dermis, which makes it rounded and smooth, deteriorates, loses some of its elastic qualities and lets down the top layer, producing the folds and wrinkles of age. The whole process happens very slowly and usually nothing is noticeable until about the 30-year-old mark, although it begins to accelerate slightly from the mid-forties onwards.*

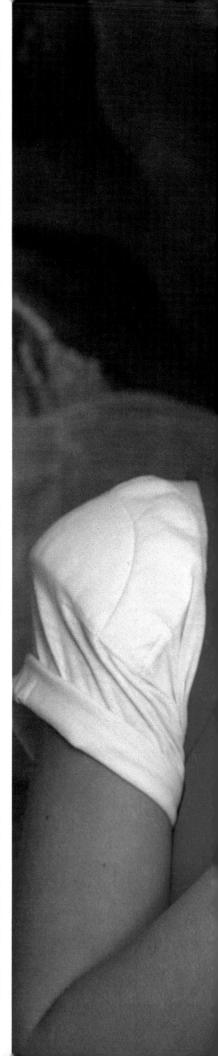

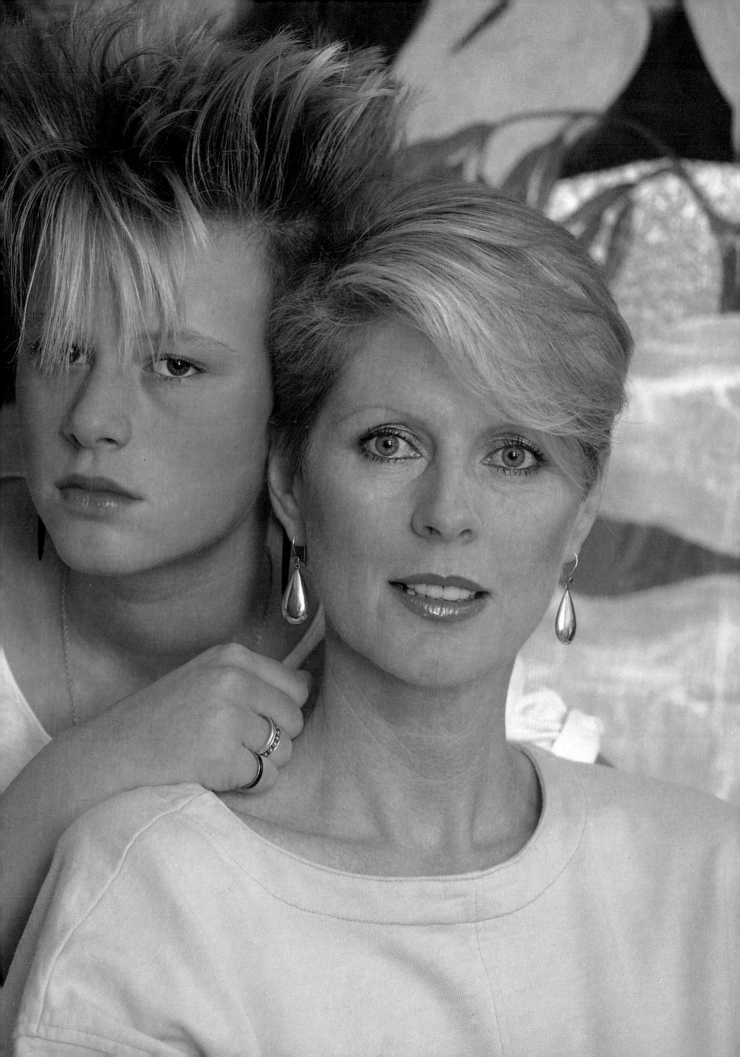

# Ageing beautifully

If you're positive about facing up to the inevitable ageing process, you're sure to keep young and enjoy life at any age. Some women look marvellous in their fifties and sixties because they have long-stay looks, the right attitude to life and are well groomed.

## Twenties

Opt for a regular gentle skin-care routine to suit your skin type. Oily skins need an oil-free skin-care range; normal to dry skins need a moisturizer. If you still suffer from outcrops of spots, choose a gentle, non-greasy cleanser and toner; confine moisturizer to dry areas (around eyes for instance) and wear a water-based foundation in an oil-free range.

## Thirties

This is when the fine lines show around eyes, between brows and sometimes from nose to jaw. Do take skin-care very seriously with meticulous cleansing, toning and moisturizing. Exposure to sun, even on a walk, must always be accompanied by a protective sun cream. Use moisturizer under make-up. Choose non-streaking powder eye-shadows and true lip colours.

## Forties

From now on, the sebacious glands slow down production; collagen fibres thin, leading to a slacker skin; the skin's ability to hold moisture diminishes. Exercise and moisturize regularly. Use light cosmetics – heavy make-up can emphasize lines. Go for powder shadows and blushers and choose matt lip shades. Outline lips with a pencil for definition. Keep out of the sun, unless you prefer brown wrinkles to slightly less deep, white ones. If you need spectacles now, wear them, it's better than squinting.

## Fifties

Wrinkles become pronounced, hair will thin a little and there are some hormonal shifts. Meticulously cleanse, moisturize skin and condition your hair. You may need a lighter shade of foundation and a lighter hair tint than your natural shade. Choose soft shades of powder shadow and blusher. Keep a clear lip-line.

## Sixties

Top-to-toe skin-care is vital, because moisture loss really sets in now. Take more time over skin-care, cleansing, toning and moisturizing. Use light-textured foundation. Keep powder eyeshadows to outer edges of eye and sweep up towards brow for a mini face-lift. Wear a neat hairstyle whether long or short; aim for flattering necklines or a pretty scarf; wear colours that add warmth to your face. Eat sensibly and be sure to exercise.

## Youthful tips

Given reasonable good health and a little luck with what you inherit, there are a few simple ways of maintaining a youthful, active body and long-lasting looks.

**Sleep** is a necessity, but it doesn't have to become an obsession. People's sleep requirements vary vastly, so as long as you feel you are well on the amount of rest you have, that's fine. Try to have the occasional afternoon nap if you tend to suffer from post-lunch fatigue, whatever your age (for more on sleep see page 169).

**A balanced diet** that promotes cell renewal, provides protection against illness and keeps your weight stable and reasonably in tune with weight-for-height chart (see page 58), is a sensible way to stay youthful and fit. Excess weight doesn't hold together so well in maturity; it can be less a matter of rounded curves, more a hint of saggy lumps. If scales show a heavier weight than you like, get rid of overmatter slowly with a good diet. The further you go past 30 the less elastic your skin becomes, so frequent and drastic weight fluctuations will result in haggard looks and flaps of superfluous skin.

Eat lots of fresh fruit and vegetables (see diet page 57), and as many as possible raw and in their skins. Over-cooking kills off many vitamins and minerals so cook quickly in a little water. In addition to the valuable fibrous intake of fruit and vegetable peel, aim for wholegrain bread, cereals, brown rice. All are more nutritious than the refined variety. They also help to waylay any tendencies towards constipation – with its consequent toxic retention – which handicaps the efficiency and appearance of the body.

See that your diet contains plenty of fish, shell fish, offal, dark-leaved vegetables, citrus fruits and all the berries, and try to maintain a daily intake of natural yogurt, honey and wheatgerm. Regular helpings of eggs and milk and cheese go without saying, but limit yourself to four eggs a week, skimmed milk and low fat cheeses if you're incined to slap on extra kilos easily or suffer from 'jodhpur' thighs. Recent tests suggest that women who retain excess fat on thighs and buttocks (even if the rest of the body is slim) have difficulty in absorbing heavy fats, so cut them down, or out, and see what happens. Drink lots of fresh and bottled water, vegetables and fruit juices – particularly apple which helps to flush out toxics. Play safe, and take a daily multi-vitamin pill to keep up the good work.

**Regular exercise** stimulates the circulation and encourages cell renewal. It aids digestion, relaxation, body suppleness, lung expansion, weight control, increases energy potential and keeps the whole body in healthy tip-top form. And it can also be very enjoyable.

Swimming utilizes practically every muscle in the body and you can take it at your own pace (see page 82). Try to fit in a couple of fun swims a week and a daily walk in the fresh air. Join a keep-fit class, take up yoga, tap-dancing, badminton or cycling . . . anything that gives you exercise with a bit of fun and preferably pleasant companions.

**Avoiding stress** which can lead to anything from nervous tension to a major illness. Stress burns up energy wastefully, throws posture disastrously, leads to shallow breathing (and a cut-back in life-enhancing oxygen) and encourages tension lines on the forehead and round the mouth.

If life consists of a whirl of activity . . . or you worry about everything from the dog's off-days to the way your children are growing up . . . or worse, you don't have enough to think about, it pays to revamp your life. Force yourself not to worry (or to worry less) about things that may never happen; take up something you enjoy and think positively about everything you do. Even the washing up can be almost a pleasure for you if you listen to your favourite record, tape or radio programme while doing it.

## Age signs

**Brown wrinkles** may look better than pasty white ones, but take care. The sun accelerates dehydration and speeds up the thinning out of the collagen layer. In other words, it leads to premature ageing. Catch your rays gently, protect your skin with a lotion that has a high sun protection factor, and guard against melanin 'spots' with a sun block. These marks – perhaps better known as liver or age spots – are caused by a slow-down in reproduction of melanin cells so the colour distribution becomes uneven. Try a medicated skin cream which

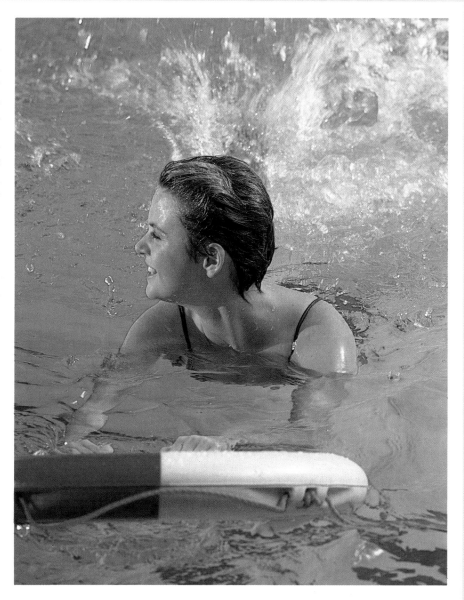

dissolves this build-up beautifully and camouflages at the same time.

**Teeth** are an important part of youthful looks. Plaque – the sticky film composed of bacteria and materials from saliva – is the major enemy. Left around the gums in hard-to-clean areas, it causes inflammation and eventually destroys the fibres that hold the teeth in place. Your dentist will get rid of hardened plaque and show you how to keep your mouth as clean as possible with brush, wooden gum massager and dental floss (see page 153).

**Eyesight** However perfect your eyesight has been, around the 40 mark your arms may no longer seem long

*Swimming is an exercise that can be enjoyed whatever your age.*

enough to let you read the newspaper in comfort. Presbyopia has set in. The lens inside the eye has become less flexible and the muscles holding it get tired of the hard work and don't do it as well as they once did.

Get yourself a super-looking pair of specs and wear them when you need to. If you already wear glasses for some eye defect, there is no need to resort to bi-focals (which are an immediate age give-away); varifocal lenses, where the prescription changes gently from bottom to top of lens with no awful dividing line, are the perfect solution.

**Varicose veins** are unsightly and often uncomfortable and they can happen even to the best regulated body. Leg veins take a heavy workload as they transport blood to and from the heart. Vein walls can weaken, sometimes resulting in a permanently knotty bulge.

Excess weight adds to the pressures; pregnancy hormones can lead to a permanent relaxation of the wall; constipation may well encourage them and there is certainly a hereditary factor involved in this condition.

The only cure in extreme cases is an operation to strip the offending vein. But prevention is better than cure. Keep your weight in order, discourage constipation, put your legs up for the occasional rest, take plenty of walks and don't wear terribly tight clothes (like waist pinching, crutch-cutting jeans). And take a look at the latest line in fashion support tights which not only look good but feel wonderfully comfortable to wear.

**Cellulite** (see page 86) which gives a puckered look to your skin, tends to sit around thighs and buttocks. While it can happen to anyone, it favours the post-30 female with a tendency to sluggish circulation and toxic retention. There is a thickening of the connective tissue and a mixture of fat, water and toxics are trapped in lumpy pockets beneath the skin. It's hard to shift but exercise helps, so do low-fat diets and lots of fresh food. Thousands of French women use kits with massage gloves, soap and creams as a regular anti-cellulite ritual in the shower or bath (see also page 161.)

**Hair** (see pages 102 to 117) gets less natural feeding from the scalp with the passing years and grey hair is more porous than natural coloured hair because the cell structure is less dense. Condition hair regularly with a rinse and give it the occasional conditioning treatment. Find a hairdresser who flatters your looks, is pleasant and will say no to any chemical processing if your hair is not in top grade health. And take his or her advice.

The menopause may bring about extra perspiration around the head. Use a gentle shampoo in a frequency range which you can use daily. As ovaries cease to function at maximum output, there may be some hair loss. It is a temporary state of affairs that will right itself, so don't panic at the sight of a little fall-out – worry only adds to the problem (see page 117).

**Late pregnancies** cause no more problems than youthful ones provided your health and muscle tones are in good order. Do every pre- and post-natal exercise in the book, act sensibly and enjoy your condition and your baby.

**Bad habits** Smoking 'kippers' the skin, kills off vitamins and leads to facial lines, so do your best to cut it out if you can or reduce numbers drastically.

Alcohol in strong doses can lead to a nasty network of broken veins and a certain amount of dehydration of the body in general. Cut out spirits and substitute the occasional glass of wine instead.

All drugs are potential sources of harm – even the domestic aspirin. A course of antibiotics prescribed by your doctor is better than four weeks with tonsillitis, but avoid any pills or medicines that aren't absolutely necessary.

**Depression** is about the most ageing thing you can have. If you can control it you'll control the totally negative effects it has on your looks and health.

But most important, don't get stuck in a rut. Be ready to try something new – from a different sort of job to an unexpected night out – or even a trip round the world! Be positive, ready to face change and enjoy life at any age. It's a sure way of keeping young.

**As you grow older . . .**
By all means colour grey hair, but lighten it gradually from the original shade. As skin lightens over the years a complementing lighter hair shade looks less artificial. If you're planning a big colour change, avoid strict partings and have regular colourings so 'seams' don't show as hair grows.

Keep upper arms in shape by standing in a doorway, hands on frame level with head. Push and relax . . . push and relax.

You'll stay looking young if you look after your spine. Stand upright, walk with a bounce and keep those vital vertebrae supple and protected. Don't slump, however tired you are – a 'tall' spine helps you to feel more full of energy.

Thighs and buttocks bear the brunt of cellulite deposits, so massage them daily. Exercise as much as possible and cultivate sensible eating habits. Drink plenty of water but little alcohol.

Walk barefoot with toes spread wide whenever possible. The basis of good balance comes from this point, so don't spoil it by teetering on over-high heels or sloppy mules.

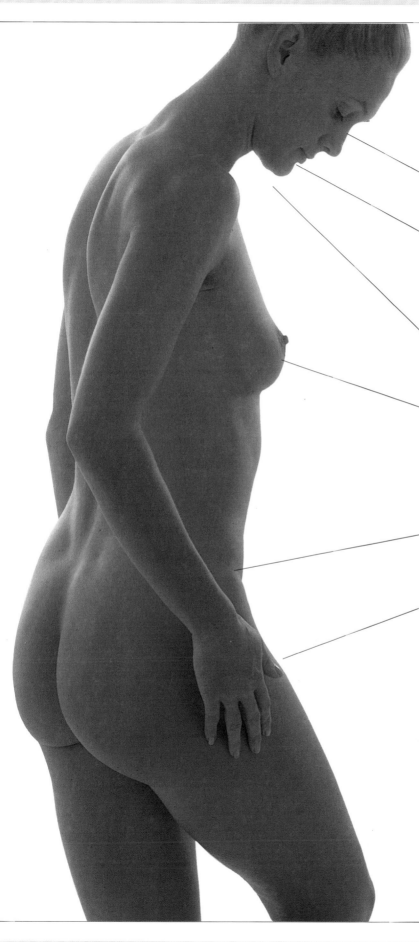

It's only too easy to develop a droop between eye and brow. Give yourself a mini facelift by tweezing away outer $\frac{1}{2}$in/1cm of brows, pencilling in replacements so that the outer edge finishes $\frac{1}{2}$in/1cm higher than your natural brow.

Presbyopia (a form of long sight) sets in at around 40, so always wear specs for close work – it's better than a frown.

Lip outlines should be perfectly crisp and clear with no trace of smudging. Outline with lip pencil, soften this line with a cotton bud and fill in very carefully with a lip brush, ensuring no little wrinkles go lipstickless.

Good posture and moisturizers help here. Exercise by holding a clenched fist under your jaw. Try to open your mouth while resisting with that fist.

If you're more than 20 years old and take a larger bra size than an A cup . . . then never go without a really well-fitting bra unless you're in bed or in water – swimming is very good for this hard-to-hold area. Pension off old bras and treat yourself to a sexy new one – try to buy with the help of a trained fitter.

Banish excess flab by smacking the stomach quite hard with the fist or your hand in swift, upward movements. Do this 20 times a day to move the bulge.

Hands age first so protect them with gloves and creams, and exercise for shape and suppleness.

# Pregnancy

There is a theory that the Mona Lisa has that marvellous enigmatic smile and looks so extraordinarily beautiful because the model was three months' pregnant when Leonardo da Vinci painted her.

Whether that is true or not, one thing certainly is true: a healthy, happy, pregnant woman undoubtedly can look her most beautiful. Her hair, her skin, everything about her glows – and it is a beauty that is not lost as the baby enlarges and changes her shape.

But – and this is important – beauty does depend to a large extent on health and happiness. A pregnant woman who is tired, lacking essential nutrients and taking inadequate care of herself will look as drab as she feels. And an unhappy woman can never look her best, whether she is pregnant or not.

## A healthy intake for two

Remember that pregnancy is not an illness. You are not in a 'delicate condition' or at risk of damage just because you're having a baby. But you do need to change your routine so that your pregnancy is what it's meant to be – a normal physiological experience.

Food matters, of course. The baby needs many of the building blocks of life for growing, and gets them only from the mother via the umbilical cord which links them. But it is the quality of your diet that counts, not the quantity.

The ideal pregnancy diet is rich in raw fruit and vegetables and whole grains; low in refined sugar and starch; adequate in protein; and fairly low in fat.

A daily helping of animal protein – meat, fish, eggs, cheese, milk – is needed, and to make sure there is not too much fat in your diet, make the protein fish or poultry more often than red meat. Grilled chicken and white fish, cottage cheese and low-fat yogurt provide excellent food without excess fat.

If you take lots of fresh raw fruit and vegetables and eat only wholemeal bread when you want bread, you'll get most of the minerals and vitamins you need. However, your doctor or midwife may suggest you take a vitamin or mineral (especially iron) supplement as well, though medical views vary on this.

As for alcohol, there is evidence that heavy and prolonged use of alcohol in pregnancy can adversely affect the growing baby, but this doesn't mean that an occasional social glass of wine or sherry can do any harm.

Smoking can result in your baby being born small and frail. Fortunately, many smokers lose their taste for cigarettes early in pregnancy (it makes them sick), and they find it fairly easy to kick the habit for good.

## Exercise in pregnancy

There is no need to give up all your normal physical activities just because you're pregnant (and that includes sex, which is an excellent form of exercise) unless a doctor specifically forbids it.

Also, the old idea that stretching, lifting or jumping can damage an unborn child is false. However, it is worth remembering that during pregnancy the joints soften a little under the influence of the hormone progesterone, and this can result in low back strain and pain.

Learning how to lift safely is an important skill to master. You should never bend down to pick up a heavy weight (for example, an older child), but bend at the knees, and squat before you begin lifting. That way you protect your back and carry the weight with the legs and other muscles which are better able to cope. Adequate rest is also needed, not because pregnancy makes you weak, but because your body is working extra hard. A daily rest in later pregnancy and time spent with your feet up give you the chance to recover your energy. Putting your feet up also helps to protect against varicose veins.

## Your changing emotions

In all the fuss that is made about a mother-to-be's physical welfare, it is possible to lose sight of the importance of psychological good health. Some women do become bothered by feelings they didn't expect and don't fully understand. Some become edgy, weepy and moody. The cause can be a mixture of physical and emotional factors: changes in hormone balance and tiredness brought on by bad eating and inadequate rest; anxiety over new responsibilities and possible changes in relationships with partner and family.

Accepting that this is common and riding out the edgy feelings helps a lot. Too often mothers-to-be get more agitated because they fret over being agitated! It helps enormously to talk about how you feel, with your partner, of course, and your doctor and/or midwife. They can be a tower of strength.

Feelings about sex may change. Some women become very amorous when they're pregnant – after all, you're never more feminine than when your uterus is doing the job it was designed for! However, other women lose some of their sex drive. Both attitudes are normal. But it is obviously essential to tell your man how you feel and to reassure him that the changes are in your body, not in your love for him.

In fact, healthy happiness during pregnancy, as at any other time, is strongly dependent on one main organ, your tongue. The more you talk about your doubts, anxieties and hopes, the better you will be able to cope . . . and to enjoy your pregnancy.

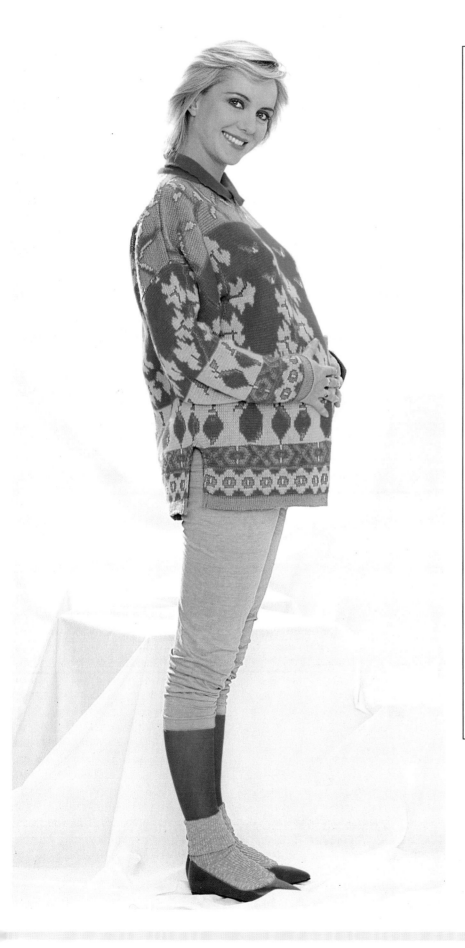

Jane Newman, former Hot Gossip dancer, gave up work when she was three months' pregnant so she could 'enjoy her pregnancy'. When we photographed her at seven months she was slim and could still do those deep pliés most of us only dream about. She borrowed Jane Fonda's *Pregnancy Workout* book from the library, decided which exercise she felt comfortable with – very important for pregnant mums – and then spent half an hour every day, stretching and building up her muscles.

One tip from Jane is: never fall out of bed and start excercising, let the body loosen up first, otherwise ligaments get torn. Yoga-based exercises helped Jane to rest her back (for her backache was the most unpleasant side-effect of pregnancy). And to help her to open her pelvis, Jane always turned upright chairs around and straddled them like an old-time cowboy.

Luckily, nature put Jane off wine, coffee and cream cakes but she was also strict with herself, allowing no over-indulgence just because she was pregnant. And for the dreaded indigestion, Jane took milk of magnesia.

This routine stood Jane in good stead when she gave birth to her baby boy.

# Cosmetic surgery

For the price of an expensive holiday abroad you can buy a facelift that will turn the clock back 10 years. Cosmetic surgery isn't reserved for the rich and famous. Thousands of ordinary men and women spend their savings at private clinics throughout the world where surgeons will remodel their looks – changing the shapes of noses, trimming ears, lifting wrinkles, slicing flab from stomach and buttocks.

For many women, cosmetic surgery offers the chance of attaining the looks they've always dreamed of. For others, it's a new lease of life. But it's a step that should not be taken lightly as undergoing cosmetic surgery usually involves big money and . . . there are risks. Here are some of the operations available.

The most popular operations for women in this booming business are facelifts, breast reductions and breast enlargments and, for men, remodelled noses and hair transplants.

Ideally, cosmetic surgery should be arranged through your doctor who, if sympathetic enough, will refer you to a cosmetic surgeon. However, it isn't always easy to persuade your doctor that you need to have that extra 6 in/15 cm on your bust, that you need your abdomen reduced, or you really don't like the shape of your nose.

In the UK surgeons cannot advertise but cosmetic surgery clinics can – and do. The trouble with most of their brochures is that they gloss over the side-effects. Face lifts don't magically happen overnight; for several weeks after the operation, you will suffer from puffiness, redness and bruising. You can cut down the lengthy stays at clinics but you certainly wouldn't be ready to face work or the world as quickly as a lot of people imagine. So,

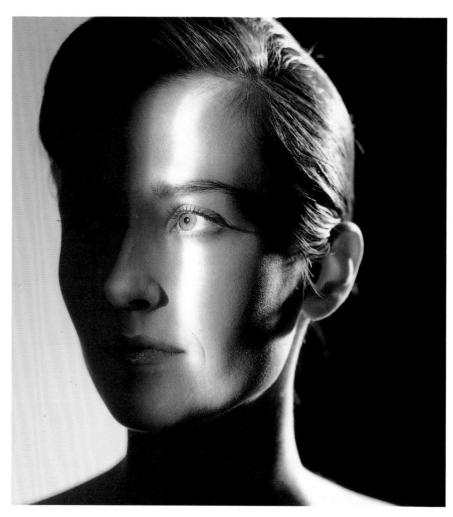

before embarking on any costly operation, make sure that you know all the medical facts. If you're going through an emotional crisis, like divorce or a split from a loved one, a facelift isn't necessarily the answer.

Consider the alternatives first: for instance, if you simply don't like the shape of your nose, try accentuating other parts of your face – make the most of your eyes or mouth (see our eye and lip tips, pages 38 and 39.)

## Facelift (Rhytidoplasty)
This falls into two categories – full facelift or the popular mini lift which is only half the face. The object of facelifts is to remove sagging facial lines prominent from the eyes down to the mouth and around the jawline. The full lift includes furrowed brow lines.

Incisions are made at the hairline

*Cosmetic surgery is a step that shouldn't be approached lightly – make sure you know the medical facts.*

near the ears and the slack skin is drawn back and up. This tightens a dropping chin line and smooths out a lot of surface lines from nose to mouth and across the chin line.

## The eyes (Blepharoplasty)
You can have both upper or lower lids lifted. It's normally the lower eyelids which need correction initially since they're the first to become puffy and wrinkled. When the bags appear, the overhanging slack skin causes a hooded effect, our eyes look tired and haggard.

Bags don't necessarily come with age – in some cases it's hereditary, along with dark circles and sagging lines. Removing the bags and lifting the eyes is often combined with a facelift. The incisions taken in the natural folds where tissue is removed leave a row of fine thread-like stitches and, in most cases, patients look slightly swollen and bruised. Not surprisingly, since the eyes are the most delicate part of the body, it can take up to six months before they 'settle' and feel normal again.

## Abdomen (*Lipectomy*)

Stomach tissue can be reduced. Sagging stomachs and bottoms can be treated surgically, and surplus fat trimmed, but this is not a popular operation since it involves fairly extensive surgery, and the patient will be scarred as a result. Flabby tissue is removed from the stomach

---

### Beat cellulite – the French way

A few years ago, a Frenchman, Dr Gerard Illouz, came up with a revolutionary surgical technique of removing fatty bulges from the body, whereby patients are left with only a tiny incision mark instead of the unsightly scarring from conventional methods.

Dr Illous operates on 'jodhpur' thighs, plump stomachs and fatty bottoms. But if you're fat all over, the Illouz technique won't do. He is only interested in the bulges.

A scalpel is used, but only to make the tiniest of incisions, then a cannula, a long curved instrument, is inserted and operates like a mini vacuum cleaner over the bulges, sucking out the fatty cells. The aim is to remove 80 per cent of the fat so that, even if a woman then puts on weight, there are no bumps.

Dr Illouz prefers his patients to be under 55 since the elasticity of the skin is better, tighter, and falls back into shape more easily.

---

with the incision made across the bikini line. For prominent buttocks, an incision will be made under the cheek and the flab drawn in.

## Breast augmentation

This is one of the more popular operations in the USA. The size of the breasts is increased by the insertion of a small bag filled with silicone gel (called a prosthesis) which is placed beneath the breast tissue, next to the rib cage. With small or sagging breasts, this bag can actually push out the existing skin, making firm up-tilted breasts with a flattering, more prominent shape.

Which size to choose? Most women are guided by their surgeons, since too-large silicone breasts could look top-heavy in relation to the rest of the figure. The operation usually involves spending three nights in a clinic; slight bruising and stiffness lasts for a couple of weeks.

This operation does not prevent you from discovering a lump in the breast, should there ever be one. Only in rare cases does the the prosthesis harden; if it does, it may have to be removed. Women whose breasts have been augmented can still breast feed.

## Breast reduction (*Mammaplasty*)

This is a major operation. It's more expensive than augmentation because of the difficulty of removing excess breast tissue. The nipple is intact, although it may have been repositioned, but breast-feeding is no longer possible. The breasts may look firmer for a time, but they will sag, as anyone's would, with age.

## Nose remodelling (*Rhinoplasty*)

There are various forms of remodelling noses. You can have a nasal bump removed, flared nostrils drawn in, a long nose shortened, a bulbous tip re-shaped, or a broad nose narrowed. In fact, if you simply don't like the shape of your nose, it can be completely redone.

This operation is often performed on car accident victims who have been thrown through the windscreen.

A lot of the alterations are carried out delicately from the inside of the nose, so there are no visible scars afterwards. The usual length of stay in a clinic is three or four nights, then the patient returns home with a plaster of paris cast over the nose for 10 days or more. It can take weeks for the swelling and bruising to settle down.

## Chin surgery (*Mentoplasty*)

Receding chins can be brought forward by means of an implant, but it may not be possible to reduce the size of a prominent chin – depending on the position of the teeth. Removing a double chin is usually done at the same time as a facelift.

## Hair transplant

There are two ways to transplant hair – the punch grafting method and the flap grafting method. The former removes hair from the back of the head in small sections, and plants it in the bald patches. Flap grafting is more difficult, since the sections of hair involved are much larger.

## Other points to consider

● Be sure that it's only vanity that makes you seek surgery. There's nothing wrong with wanting to get rid of the untidy wrinkles of age or a badly misshapen feature, but don't have your looks altered just because you are generally depressed and think you might feel better mentally if your nose or jawline were changed.

● Be totally sure it is what you want and willing to bear the cost, the inconvenience and discomfort you will have to put up with.

● Don't worry that everyone will immediately think: 'She's had a nose-job, or a breast or facelift.' Most people who see you after successful cosmetic surgery will just think you're looking better.

# Beauty from Within

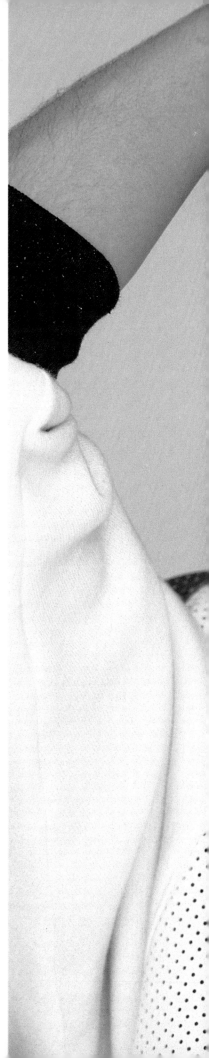

*A woman's attitude to herself conditions her appearance far more than cosmetics or expensive surgery could ever do. If you feel good, you are likely to look good (and vice versa!) and to function better both at work and at play.*

*It's a well-known fact that three times more women than men visit their doctor with minor nervous disorders whose symptoms include: feelings of isolation and inadequacy, lapses of concentration and memory, constant fatigue, crying, over-eating or under-eating, feelings of guilt, and insomnia.*

*In this chapter we examine the causes of some of these symptoms and offer advice on how to combat them by reorganizing your lifestyle and relaxation techniques. There are also practical tips for keeping in tip-top form both mentally and physically – and a guide to self-help health to minimize the risk of contracting diseases such as breast or cervical cancer, and heart problems.*

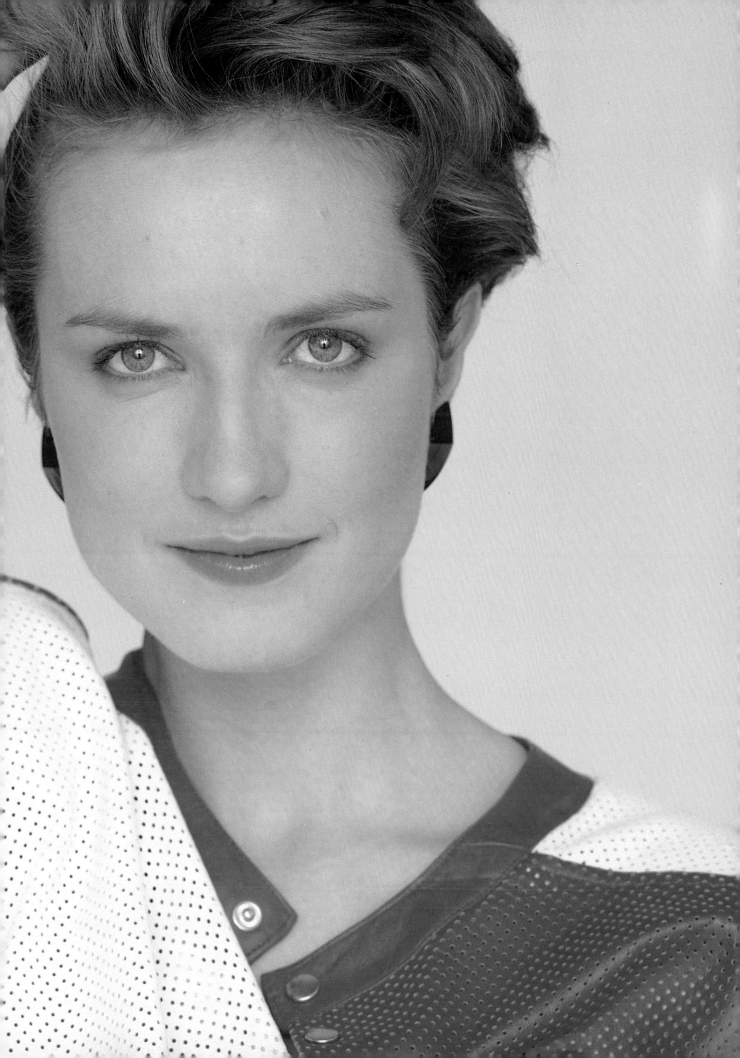

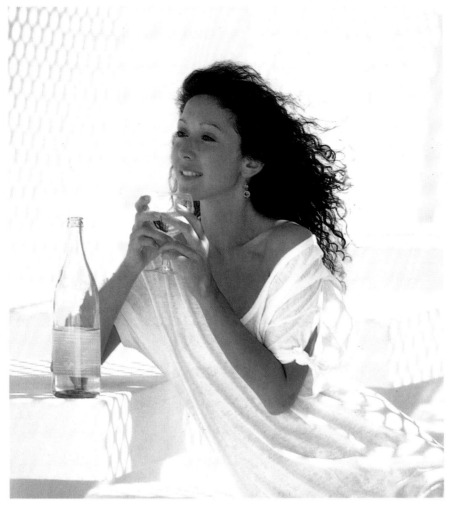

## Keep healthy and happy

Here are 25 simple tips to put you on the road to health and happiness.

**1** Eat lots of fresh fruit and vegetables, wholemeal bread and whole bran breakfast foods to make your digestive system more efficient.

**2** Reduce the amount of meat you eat, making sure that the meat you do eat is cooked properly.

**3** Reduce the amount of animal fat in your diet.

**4** Eat sugary foods only at mealtimes and then in moderation.

**5** Drink no more than 2½ pints/1·4 litres of beer or five small glasses of wine or five single spirits – preferably diluted – per day. If you are pregnant, restrict yourself to two glasses of wine.

*Drink plenty of water each day to cleanse the system, and try to follow our 25 pointers to a healthier way of life.*

**6** Brush your teeth at least twice a day and, ideally, after meals too. Use a soft-bristled, small-headed toothbrush and brush with a circular movement. Pay particular attention to gum margins.

**7** Use dental floss or soft wooden tooth picks to clean between your teeth.

**8** Buy an electric toothbrush to help to prevent the gum disease periodontitis.

**9** Eat a small piece of hard cheese after meals. The calcium in cheese is good for teeth.

**10** Make sure you take adequate relaxation whenever possible in whatever way appeals to you, but balance it with exercise as well.

**11** Try to get out in the fresh air whenever possible, especially in the winter.

**12** If you don't already take regular exercise, begin now.

**13** Go for a brisk 20-minute walk at least three times a week and/or a 20-minute swim. But remember if you're not used to exercise, don't overdo it at first.

**14** Providing you are medically fit, try to do something strenuous every day that makes you out of breath.

**15** Put all your major joints – hips, knees, shoulders – through their full range of movements at least once a day.

**16** Join an exercise class. Regular stretching exercises tone up the muscles and help to keep your body supple.

**17** Have a cervical smear test once a year, especially if you are over 35.

**18** Check in good time before you go abroad that all your vaccinations are up to date.

**19** All women of childbearing age should be immunized against German measles (rubella).

**20** Give up smoking.

**21** If you intend to become pregnant, stop smoking. If you continue to smoke your baby is likely to be lighter and less healthy.

**22** From the moment you know you are pregnant, pay attention to all health points.

**23** Stick to a regular bedtime, bearing in mind that two hours 'sleep before midnight are worth four afterwards.

**24** If you are around 35 and glaucoma runs in the family, have your eyes checked.

**25** If you're lonely, don't wait for someone to get in touch with you. Phone or write to a friend.

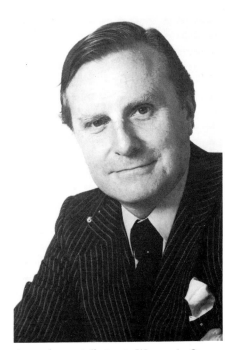

*A regular contributor to* Woman's Own, *Dr Mike Smith is a specialist in community medicine, chief medical officer of The Family Planning Association and broadcaster. Here's his advice on how to avoid stress.*

# Stress

When our ancestors had to fight for survival or flee from wild animals or enemies, stress, caused by fear, was actually a good thing because it prepared their bodies for action. Today, however, stress can be caused by many, not necessarily life-threatening, factors and, lacking immediate outlets, often turns in on itself. That's when the trouble begins. Learn to recognize when you're under stress and, more importantly, how to take life more calmly and feel happier as a result.

Joy and excitement, as well as fear and worry, can cause stress. When you fall in love, for instance, you may find you have trembling hands, fast-beating heart and tension in the stomach when you catch sight of your loved one.

## What causes stress symptoms?

Depending on the degree and urgency of the excitement or fear, an increase in electrical activity occurs in our nerves and the concentration of stress-released hormones in our blood. We go clammy as our sweat glands work hard to cool us, we look pale and we feel 'butterflies' in our stomach as blood is diverted away from our skin and intestines to our muscles.

Whenever possible, these stress-charged events (see box) should be spaced out so that you have time to adjust. It is very important to determine your own pace.

If your house is on fire you naturally want to get out as soon as possible. Under such stress, the muscles, heart and lungs respond instantly to the impulses passed through the automatic (reflex) nervous system and only a little more slowly to the hormones – adrenalin and hydrocortisone, for instance – from the adrenal glands. The result is an increase in muscle tone, heart-rate, blood pressure and breathing.

The brain becomes alert, too, as energy foods – sugars – are released into the bloodstream from the liver, fuelling both the brain and body. The stores of fatty energy are also mobilized, increasing the blood's fat concentration.

The increased rate of the heart beat allows it to pump the sugar-rich blood around the body faster. It also carries extra oxygen, which is being inhaled faster by deep, quick breathing. Without oxygen, the sugar can't produce energy. More blood cells (platelets, responsible for the blood's clotting) are then produced. These together with other components of the blood play an important part in healing wounds should we be injured.

All these things are useful if you're in training for, say, a marathon or some equally important athletic event. In the short term, they help you to get the best out of yourself.

## Long-term dangers

In the long term, however, the bodily changes caused by stress may result in real disease. Sustained high stress levels causing the release of fats and clotting platelets in the blood may, for example, cause heart attacks. High stress levels can also cause high blood pressure which, in turn, can contribute to other types of heart and kidney disease and strokes.

The manifestations of stress are many and varied. Headache, neck, shoulder and back pain sufferers may find stress to be the cause, as may those who complain of 'butterflies' in the stomach, palpitations or a frequent desire to pass urine.

Other stress-related disorders include chronic constipation, diarrhoea, skin rashes, peptic ulcers, excessive sweating, menstrual and sexual problems, insomnia (see page 170) and irritability.

Any of these conditions are likely to be aggravated by over-eating, drinking or smoking.

## Those most at risk

The executive who can sort out a preferred work pattern and priorities, take holidays when desired and delegate work that doesn't demand personal attention, is unlikely to suffer from stress diseases, even though the responsibilities and apparent reasons for stress may be great.

| Your stress-point chart | |
|---|---|
| | Stress |
| *Unhappy events* | points |
| Death of a spouse | 100 |
| Divorce | 73 |
| Marital separation | 65 |
| Imprisonment | 63 |
| Death of a close relative or friend | 63 |
| *Happy events* | |
| Marriage | 50 |
| Pregnancy | 40 |
| Buying a house | 31 |
| Christmas | 12 |

It's more often the over-ambitious person who never seems to have time to take a holiday, whose pace of work is constant and unrelenting, in whom the problems of stress arise. And, as the tension can't be released by fighting or fleeing, the body produces symptoms instead.

### Learn to relax the yoga way

Yoga may be just the thing to help you to relax. Professionally-run classes are the best way to start. There are also plenty of books on the subject – but if you're not attending a class, take care not to try anything too difficult or strenuous at first. Relaxation and meditation classes are also good for freeing both mind and body from tension.

Yoga is an old-age form of physical *and* mental exercise that can be practised by anyone at any age. It provides the perfect 'total' exercise whether you are seemingly super-fit, pregnant, horribly out of condition or indeed if you have some medical problem or disability (provided you go to the right class and have a skilled teacher).

The mystic aspect of yoga is rarely emphasized in the Western world and the Hatha Yoga classes on offer are likely to be – at least in the early stages – primarily a physical experience. You will practise asanas or postures which exercise and balance the body, tone and stretch muscles, joints and ligaments. They will improve your circulation, work on glands, nerves, your respiratory system and internal organs.

Yoga also encourages you to make full use of your respiratory system as you learn to breathe properly during postures and progress to yoga breathing exercises or pranayama. Lessons end (and sometimes start) with a relaxation session which releases tension in the body and rests your entire system.

Although the meditative aspects are not a prominent feature of yoga teaching in this country, most people who take it up and practice regularly become aware of a change in their mental state – with in-

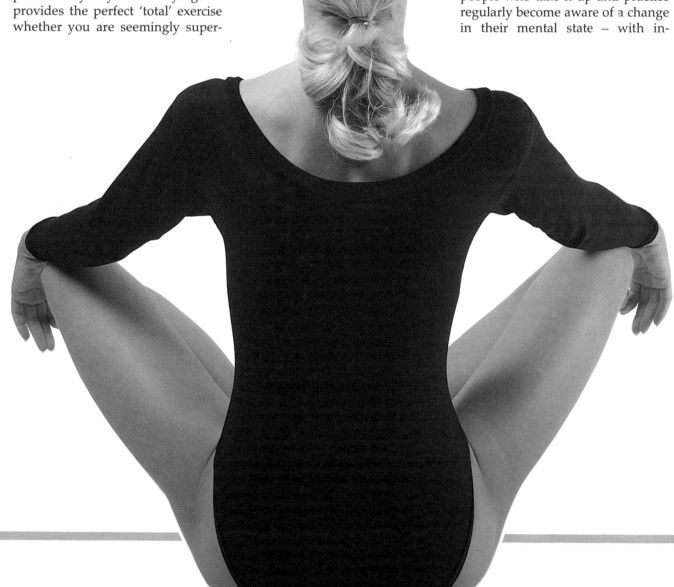

creased confidence, powers of concentration and peace of mind.

Equipment is minimal. You need only a small amount of floor space and some comfortable clothes you can move in – tights, a leotard or T-shirt – and a blanket for floor exercises and covering yourself during relaxation sessions.

It is important to work, or certainly learn, with a teacher and then to do some yoga every day to achieve the full benefits. As well as the many local authority classes all over the UK, The Yoga for Health Foundation has 80 venues for classes in Britain and a centre at Ickwell Bury, Northill, Biggleswade, Bedfordshire where they run yoga activities all through the year. In addition to normal yoga training courses, specific courses to train yoga teachers in remedial yoga are available and they now have more than 120 accredited remedial teachers of yoga including some doctors and other para-medical people. These – and the specific courses at the centre – have had great success with people suffering from chronic back problems, multiple sclerosis, Parkinson's disease and severe stress-related problems.

**Tension-easing exercises** Sit in an armchair or lie on a bed. See that the room is warm, quiet, and there are no bright lights. Breathe regularly, slowly and deeply. This alone is relaxing, especially the breathing apect.

Concentrate on one word (also called a 'mantra') to clear the mind, constantly repeating the word (try 'calm') each time you breathe out.

Lying flat on your back, clench your toes, making your calf muscles contract so you can feel the tension. Then relax and appreciate the difference – the muscles feel warm and pleasant instead of taut and uncomfortable. Do the same with your thighs, abdomen, chest, hands, arms, face and forehead. After that, concentrate on how relaxed and warm each part of your body feels. Go to sleep if it happens naturally, even if you have been told to stay awake.

Don't expect immediate results: it may be some time before you feel properly relaxed from using these techniques.

---

### How to prevent stress

● **Do** eat a well-balanced diet containing plenty of whole-meal bread, fresh fruit and vegetables.

● **Don't** make too many big changes in your life at once unless you are forced to. Make important decisions as quickly as possible; uncertainty is a potent cause of stress.

● **Do** remember that the 'props' to combat stress can aggravate rather than relieve stress. Giving up smoking and keeping other stimulants in check may actually remove the symptoms of stress.

● **Don't** be over-ambitious – ambitions are healthy only when there is some possibility of realising them.

● **Do** set aside at least half an hour for yourself each day. Just sitting quietly with feet up can do the trick. And a regular bedtime an hour before midnight seems to provide more valuable sleep (see page 170) than retiring later.

● **Don't** bottle up stress. Use exercise to let off steam. Avoid noisy environments if possible as tension caused by a noisy office can use up to 20 per cent of a person's energy.

● **Do** have a hobby. Gardening, for instance, is a stress-free channel, for the energies of the stress-prone.

---

## Sleep

Although we spend, on average, eight out of every 24 hours sleeping – that's a third of our lives – until the mid-1970s very little was known about sleep. Now, research using volunteers in sleep laboratories is enabling scientific measurements to be made. These measurements, together with the sleepers' own assessments of 'what sort of night they have had' is helping the sleep scientists to understand the nature of 'brain' sleep and how important it is for our mental and physical well-being.

### Sleep patterns
Research shows that there's quite a normal variation around a seven-and-a-half-hour average. Some people, often the more intelligent, only need to sleep for three or four hours a night. Sleep requirements differ, too, at different ages.

Babies spend much of their early days asleep and gradually increase the amount taken at night and diminish their daytime need, until they are about four years old. They continue to need more sleep than an adult, but in diminishing amounts until they reach the age of 20. The elderly will have 'fragmented' sleep but generally sleep longer overall when daytime naps are taken into account. Women in early pregnancy will sleep long and soundly, but their sleep will often be more disturbed in later pregnancy.

When you are asleep, your body is resting, but your brain is still quite active, although you are unaware of it. The brain's activity can be measured by the electroencephalograph – the EEG. When tiny electically sensitive wires are held in contact with the top of the head and connected to the EEG, a continuous recording can be kept of the sleeper's brain waves. Different wave patterns are recorded at different levels of sleep. In healthy sleep, these occur at regular intervals throughout the night.

Body movements can also be recorded by means of the electroculograph – the EOG machine. This measures the movement of the eyes under the sleeper's closed lids. Periods of rapid eye movement (REM) occur in a regular time pattern during sleep, taking place about five times each night. These periods of 20 minutes or so of REM are important because they indicate the quality of sleep.

For instance, during a night's sleep after which the average good sleeper awakes refreshed, the sleep will have followed a certain pattern throughout the night. At first, sleep will have been at the deepest level, level four, then as the night wore on, it will have risen to the next level, three, and then level two. These levels can be observed in the sleeper both by the wave tracings of the EEG machine, recording the brain's electrical measurements, and by the EOG, recording body measurements.

The old wives' tale that an hour before midnight is worth two after is, in part, substantiated by new research. It's in that first hour of healthy sleep that we reach the first of our deep sleep phases. We reach another one about two hours later. Research shows that the best time to go to bed is from 10pm to 11pm as it is then that the night's sleep will follow its normal pattern.

It's during the deep, level-four sleep, that the susceptible will walk and/or talk, and others will wet the bed. Children experience more deep level-four sleep than adults and are therefore more susceptible to these phenomena.

**Dreams** The REM phase is the time when dreaming occurs. Some sleepers will insist they don't dream, but it's more likely they don't remember. It is thought that we remain mentally healthy by dreaming during our sleep.

Nightmares may also occur during REM sleep. These bad dreams are associated with fright symptoms occurring at the same time in the body. The heart races, the sufferer sweats and muscles tighten with fear. Reassurance that all is well is what is required. When nightmares are frequent, an emotionally upsetting time or event may be the reason.

## Beauty sleep
During sleep, our bodies secrete more growth hormone which is responsible, in full-grown adults, for stimulating the continued growth of each new layer of skin (it really is beauty sleep!) and other growing tissues like hair, or the lining of the bowel, which have to be regularly replaced. It promotes the healing of scars, so wounds heal more rapidly during sleep. These repetitive processes of the body don't stop altogether when we don't sleep, but when next we do sleep, these processes will speed up to compensate for any previous delay.

## Sleep disturbances
Our sleep requirement is ordered by a process that works like a built-in clock, but it can also be influenced by our own wishes, such as when we go out on night shift or go dancing all night. Also, when the daylight hours alter slowly with the seasons, our awake and asleep timetable may vary with them, but our sleep is affected little in quantity or quality.

However, if we fly in a plane and cross time zones quickly, our clock gets confused; the sudden change is not anticipated, our biorhythm is upset and, in turn, our sleep. For several days, until we become acclimatized to the new time pattern, our sleep can be disturbed, as can our daytime mental and physical performance.

## Insomnia
These same disturbances, but with

anxiety and worry added, are the basis of insomnia. Chronic insomnia can be a symptom of mental and, less commonly, physical disease. Depression, anxiety, schizophrenia are mental examples and thyrotoxicosis (an overworking of the thyroid gland) is a physical one. But, four out of five instances of insomnia have an emotional cause.

---

### Tips for a good sleep

Here are some old and tried remedies for sleeplessness:

● Relax by taking at least 20 minutes' brisk but comfortable walk early in the day.

● Unwind an hour or so before going to bed with a warm, milky drink.

● Don't drink stimulants – coffee, tea or alcohol – before going to bed.

● Make sure the bedroom is properly ventilated – leave a window open in summer and a door slightly ajar in winter.

● Choose warm but light bedding and a bedroom temperature of about 18·5C/65F.

● Relax in a comfortably hot bath before going to bed.

● Establish, if possible, a regular bedtime before 11pm.

● Remember that a satisfying sex life is a good sleep inducer.

---

If you've tried all these remedies and are still suffering from an unexplained change in your usually satisfying sleep pattern after several days, the diagnosis of insomnia may be appropriate. This means that you'll probably be taking more than 30 minutes to fall asleep, then

**Right:** *A good night's sleep is a beauty bonus, so try to relax before going to bed.*

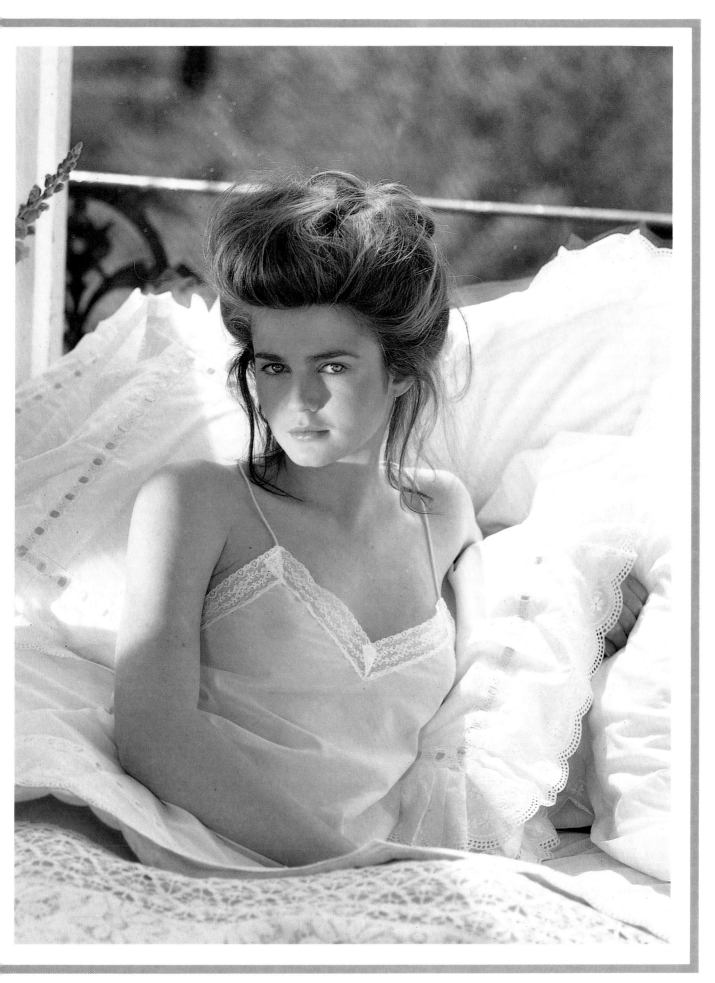

constantly waking up or waking for good one or more hours earlier than usual.

The effects of several consecutive sleeplessness nights upon the brain include making the sufferer irritable, lethargic and even altering aspects of the personality; lack of sleep can cause aggression or moroseness in someone who is naturally the opposite. The body, too, can be affected.

If you suffer from any worrying sleep disturbance, check with your doctor. But bear in mind that the sleeping pill that he or she may prescribe should be regarded only as a very short-term measure. Hangovers' from pills can be experienced the next day, affecting your mood and performance. The beneficial effects, too, often wear off after a few days. When taken for longer periods, sleeping pills can

cause 'rebound' insomnia. That is, a sufferer who stops taking them sleeps less well than before, so takes more. It's a vicious circle. Be prepared to experience lack of concentration and slowness of movement and reaction times while trying to come off the drug. You may also feel sick or actually be sick, and have considerable feelings of anxiety.

When you know you are well, and feel generally happy, but your sleep is not as good or as long as other people's appears to be, the best thing to do is to accept it. We know there are those who are larks and work best in the morning, or owls who work best late at night, but there are also many other types of perfectly normal sleep patterns.

*A three minute session with a skipping rope is a simple way of exercising at home.*

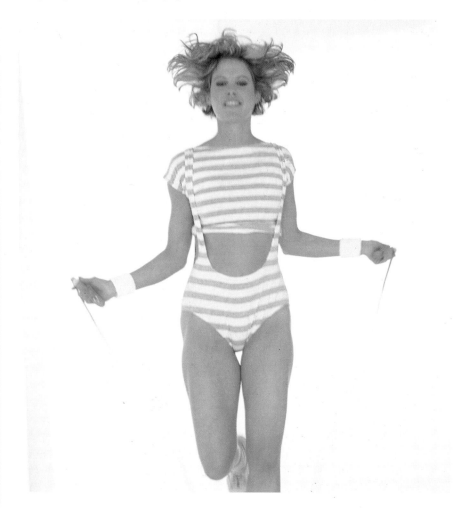

# The facts about fatigue

Most of us have at some time woken up in the morning still feeling exhausted. Although our natural reaction is to question the quality and quantity of the sleep we are having, there are other possible causes of fatigue.

Fatigue is a common symptom of anaemia, but anaemia rarely occurs unless the blood is down to about half strength. It is seldom this low. Mild anaemia is, however, common in women. On occasions the symptoms of tiredness will be attributed to the mild anaemia discovered by a blood test, simply because nothing else can be discovered to be at fault. The doctor will question and examine the person to rule out a hidden infection, painful inflammation of the joints, a malfunctioning thyroid gland, or rarely, a life-threatening condition. When the doctor finds nothing physically wrong he or she is faced with the far more difficult problem of diagnosing the cause for the tiredness in the patient's lifestyle or emotions.

Sometimes a little planning can make all the difference. The busiest people are often the least tired because they plan their day, week, even year in advance. They don't end up tired, with jobs half finished or less than well done because their schedule includes adequate break and relaxation to recharge their batteries.

### Diet '
Slimmers, especially young ones, will often complain of tiredness and find it difficult to accept that their crank, crash diet is the cause. At the other extreme, consuming too many calories makes you obese and therefore tired because you are carrying a lot of extra weight. Also, heavy fatty meals slow down the digestion. This makes you feel lethargic and much more prone to after-dinner naps.

Increasing the amount of fresh vegetables and fruit in your diet and reducing the proportion of fat and sugar can often dramatically improve your energy output, zest for life, skin appearance, and bowel action.

## Exercise

Another important factor is exercise in the fresh air. Sitting at work and on public transport in smoky, germ-filled air is a major reason why so many women think they lack energy. They overlook their need to have regular exercise and to expand their lungs. You need as little as half-an-hour's vigorous walk three times a week, although it's better still if you can manage one every day.

Many schools of relaxation advocate deep regular breathing as a means of acquiring energy and tranquillity. Vigorous walking on a regular basis will help to achieve these goals.

## Unhappiness

Dissatisfaction can produce tiredness, apathy and even despair. Worry, anxiety and negative attitudes can go on to cause mental and physical illness.

At work, we require the stimulation of goals. We need to be appreciated both for ourselves and our work. At home, we need all those things and a little more. We need to love and be loved, and to be able to afford to live in reasonable comfort and privacy.

Deprived permanently of these necessities, most human beings will eventually suffer from fatigue. We may even become mentally depressed – a real cause of sleep disturbance – and require treatment for that before we start to feel better.

# Guide to self-help health

Being fit in mind, body and spirit is often called *positive health*. Only you can achieve it for yourself. The three fundamentals for good health are: eating a balanced diet, taking appropriate exercise, and avoiding known risks like smoking cigarettes and drinking alcohol to excess. It is also up to you to arrange regular medical check-ups for various potential ills. These include:

**Breast examination** (You should do this yourself every month just after your period has finished or, if postmenopausal, on the first day of each calendar month.) Stand straight and unclothed before a mirror so that you can see both your breasts. Look for any unusual lumps or moles that have changed in size, shape or colour. Both nipples should be examined and there should be no unusual discharge. Then, lie on your back on a bed and feel both breasts with the flat of your hand. Using the right hand for the left breast and the left hand for the right breast, feel the centre of the breasts, then the lower left quarter, the lower right, the top right and the top left. After this, each armpit should be felt to ensure there are no unusual swellings. If anything unusual is found, a doctor's examination should be sought without delay. Fortunately, for as many as nine out of 10 such lumps that are found by self-examination, a doctor is able to be reassuring – but the early consultation can be vital.

**Cervical smear** This should be performed every three years up to the age of 35 and every five years thereafter. This is to detect the presence of abnormal cells on the cervix which may turn cancerous, and if caught in time, can be completely eradicated.

**Blood pressure reading** This should be taken once every three years up to the age of 35 and every year thereafter. If you smoke, are overweight, pregnant, diabetic or on the Pill, it should be taken frequently whatever your age. High blood pressure can contribute to heart disease; low blood pressure is rarely a problem.

**Dental check-up** Teeth and gums should be checked every six months and at the beginning of pregnancy for signs of tooth decay and gum disease. Teeth should be scaled and cleaned professionally at least once a year to remove plaque which calcifies and hardens on the teeth and can cause gum disease leading to eventual loss of teeth.

**Sight testing** For those with sight defects this should be done about once a year; others will require a sight test between the ages of 40 and 50 when long-sightedness may set in, plus an investigation for signs of cataract.

---

### Hints to fight fatigue

If you suffer from fatigue, use the following pointers to make your own lifestyle diagnosis before seeking medical help:

● Is your life chaotic? Are you trying to do too much and leaving many tasks half-finished? Programme your lifestyle by planning in advance – you may even get more done.

● Are you eating too much carbohydrate and not enough fruit and vegetables?

● Do you worry unduly and falsely about your 'lack of sleep'?

● Is your job a satisfying one? Are you appreciated at work?

● If your problem at home is insoluble, what do you need to do to put it right? If you can't solve the problem, can you accept it? It may then cease to cause undue anxiety.

# Health Farms

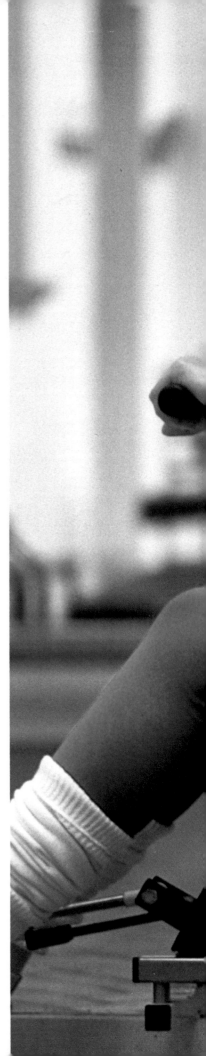

*Until the mid-1980s, the common view was that health farms were for three kinds of people: the idle rich recovering from Christmas over-indulgence, ageing actors and actresses getting into shape for their next role and health freaks. Today, the truth is that they attract people from all walks of life. Many of them go to unwind from the stresses of modern living rather than just to lose weight.*

*People who haven't been to a health farm before are naturally curious about what it's really like. To answer the most frequently asked questions, come with* Woman's Own *to one of England's most established health centres.*

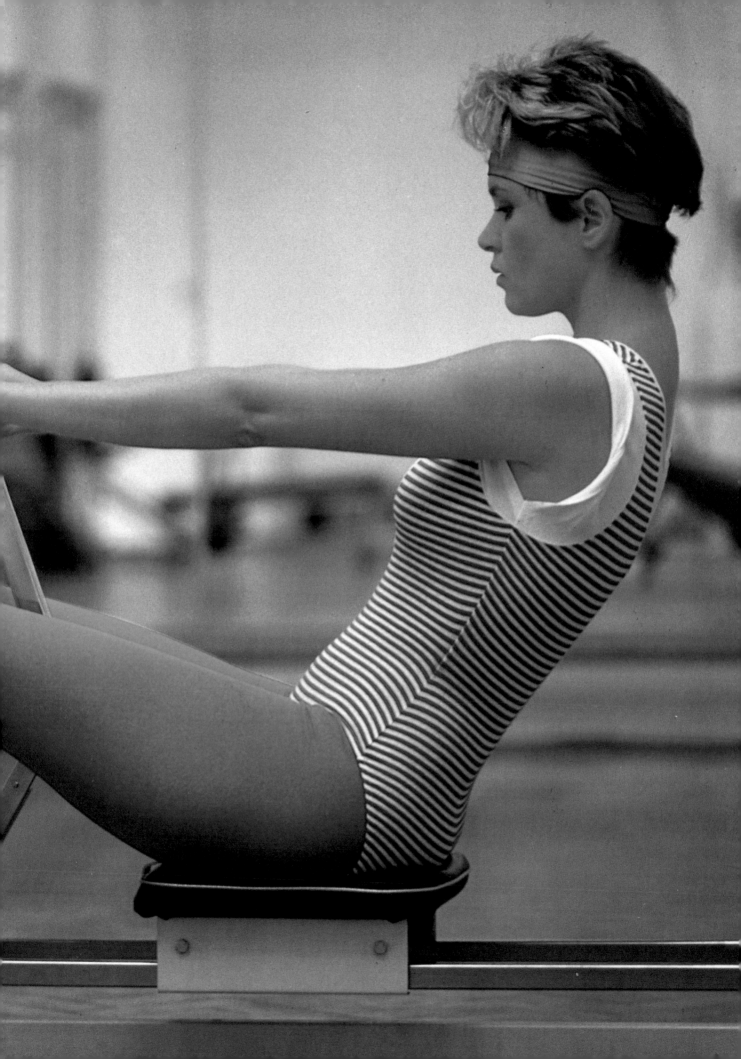

*Grayshott Hall is set in beautiful parkland (right). The public rooms are quietly luxurious and the bedrooms are pretty and comfortable. There is a magnificent swimming pool, well-equipped gymnasium (see previous page), spacious treatment rooms, a boutique and a hairdressing salon.*

## What should you pack?

Very little, is the answer. During the day, between treatments, most people live in towelling robes or track suits. Other essentials include flip-flops or terry towelling mules, leotard and tights or comfortable shorts and T-shirts for exercise classes, ballet pumps or soft lace-up shoes, track shoes or comfortable flatties for walks. In the evenings, you might want to change for dinner so take a comfortable dress or pretty shirt and skirt. Don't forget a swimsuit and – since it seems one spends half the time showering after treatments or a swim – a really large bottle of body moisturizing lotion. Newspapers and books are on sale, but you may want to take along your own reading matter – there's lots of lovely leisure time to catch up on reading.

## What will it cost?

Approximately the same as it would for a week in a luxury hotel. All meals are included in the cost, plus lots of extras: a consultation on arrival and departure to discuss weight and health problems; a massage and a steam treatment every day; exercise and yoga classes; pool exercises; evening entertainments. You pay extra for beauty treatments, hairdressing, and body-toning treatments such as G5 and Slendertone (see page 180).

## Will you be starved?

Hardly! The aim is to give your body a rest from bad eating habits, help you to lose weight and re-educate your taste buds towards deliciously healthy, nutritious food.

Here's a general diet plan offered by Grayshott Hall: when you wake up, you'll be served either hot water

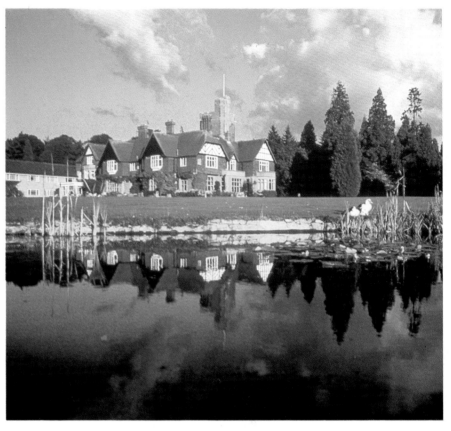

---

**Cauliflower au gratin**
(135 CALORIES)
*or*
**Avocado and orange salad**
(60 CALORIES)

**Turbon of sole 'Veronique'**
*Olives of sole with a grape and salmon mousse filling and a light fish sauce*
A selection of vegetables
(275 CALORIES)
*or*
**Grilled calf's liver**
*Served with a kumquat sauce*
A selection of vegetables
(345 CALORIES)

**Spicy fruit salad**
(65 CALORIES)
*or*
**Fruit basket**
(AVERAGE 15 CALORIES
per oz/25 g)
*or*
**A selection of cheese**
(85-115 CALORIES per oz/25 g)

A typical menu for dinner at
Grayshott Hall

---

or lemon water.

Breakfast (which is served in your room) can be fresh fruit with milk or yogurt; boiled egg with one or two crispbreads and butter and an apple; fruit juice or half a grapefruit. (If you wanted to go on a strict diet, then it would be breakfast number three – otherwise, they're alternated.) At 11 am fruit or vegetable juices are served.

Lunch is a large mixed salad served with cold fish, grated Cheddar cheese, hardboiled egg, nuts, plus two crispbreads, butter, followed by a sweet of yogurt, junket or honey-sweetened stewed fruit. (The salads are really delicious and imaginative and you can take home a list of salad suggestions to keep up the good work!) At 4 pm it's time for a cup of Chinese tea and before you know it, it's 6 pm and time to meet in the drawing room for a glass of low-calorie fruit punch.

**Right:** *You certainly won't starve at a health farm – just look at this choice of appetizing and healthy dishes!*

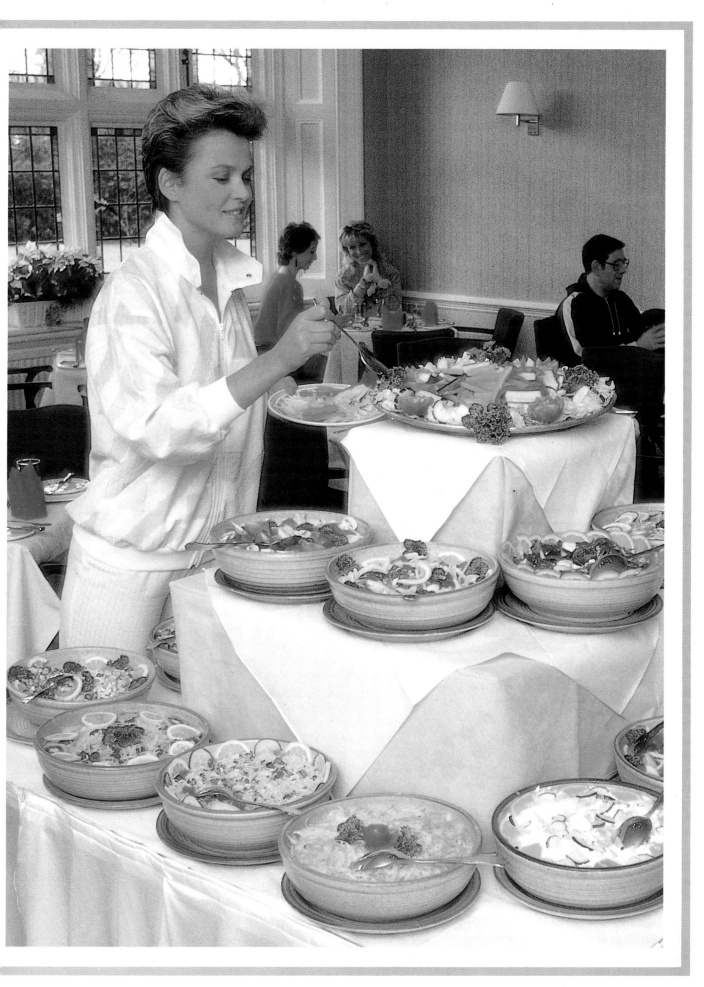

Dinner is served at 6.30 pm (see sample menu) but if you're on a strict diet for a few days, then you have the salad lunch (no sweet) and fruit or yogurt in the evening. To make it easier, there's a light diet room, so you don't have to watch the others tucking into their dinner!

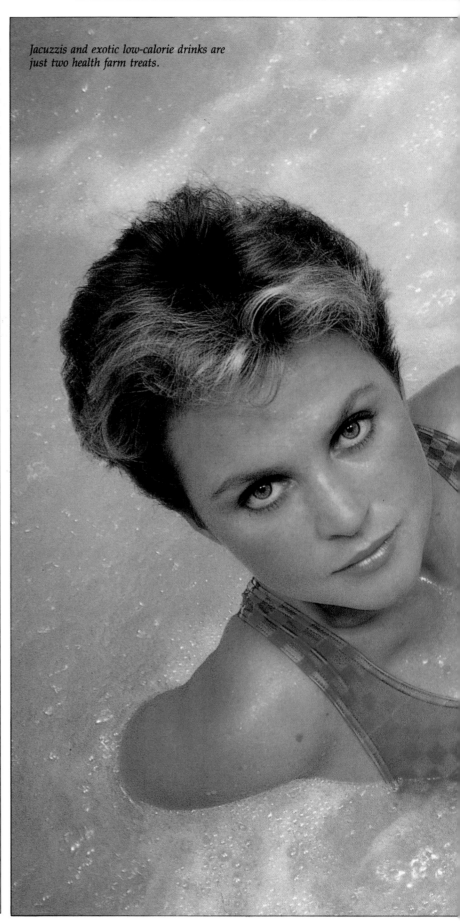

*Jacuzzis and exotic low-calorie drinks are just two health farm treats.*

## Thirty salad suggestions to try at home

Lettuce
Red cabbage, diced apple and sultanas
Sweetcorn, celery, beetroot, vinaigrette
Cucumber, asparagus, pimento, curry powder
Diced beetroot
Sliced cucumber
Crudités
Chopped peppers and onions
Grated carrot, cheese and sultanas
Brown rice, pimentoes, prawns and nuts
Watercress and Brazil nuts
Coleslaw
Salad niçoise
Russian salad
Red cabbage, lettuce and vinaigrette
Egg and onion
Grapefruit mint and mushrooms
Courgettes, apple and vinaigrette
French beans and mint
Cauliflower, cheese and tomato
Tomato slices
Sweetcorn
Mushroom and lemon juice
White cabbage, peaches and nuts
Salad Waldorf
Mustard and cress
Carrot and dates
Chicory and orange
Curried rice, pimentoes, yogurt and asparagus
Tomato, onion and vinaigrette

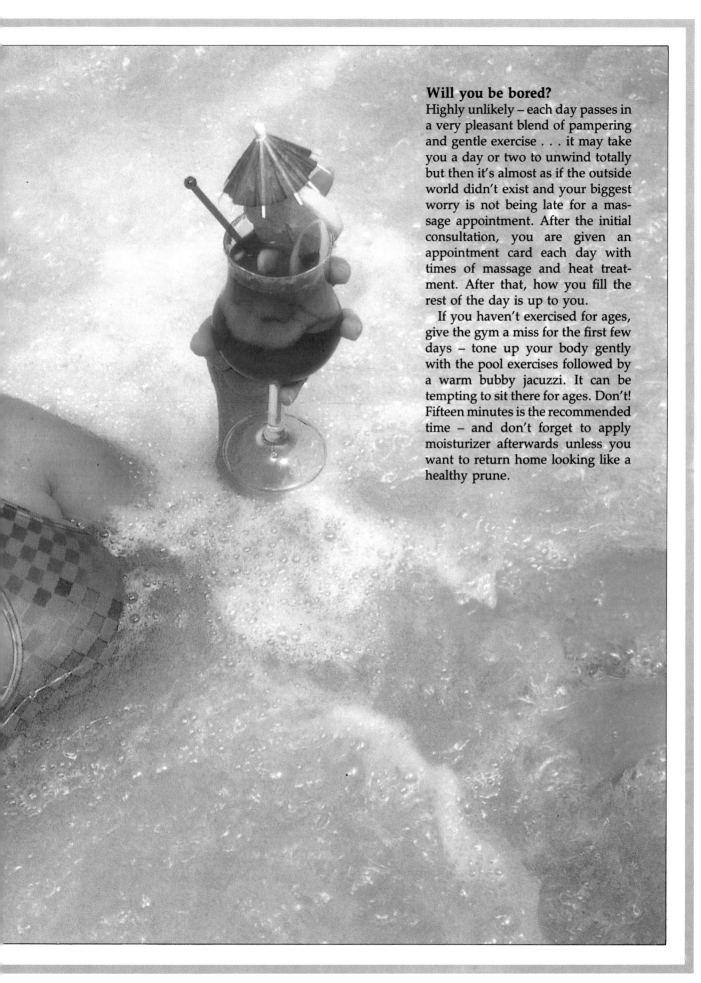

### Will you be bored?

Highly unlikely – each day passes in a very pleasant blend of pampering and gentle exercise . . . it may take you a day or two to unwind totally but then it's almost as if the outside world didn't exist and your biggest worry is not being late for a massage appointment. After the initial consultation, you are given an appointment card each day with times of massage and heat treatment. After that, how you fill the rest of the day is up to you.

If you haven't exercised for ages, give the gym a miss for the first few days – tone up your body gently with the pool exercises followed by a warm bubby jacuzzi. It can be tempting to sit there for ages. Don't! Fifteen minutes is the recommended time – and don't forget to apply moisturizer afterwards unless you want to return home looking like a healthy prune.

Why not treat yourself to a G5 or Slendertone body-toning treatment? These are available at most health farms. G5 or vibro massage is a strong mechanical form of massage for improving the circulation and helping to eliminate waste products through the lymphatic system. It is particularly effective for reducing heavy hips, thighs and large or low-slung buttocks and in tightening a slack stomach and slimming a thick midriff.

Slendertone or faradism is the name given to muscle contraction treatments whereby various types of currents are used to stimulate natural exercise. A reduction of inches may result, but it does not alter body weight unless combined with a diet.

There are organized walks each day – or you can borrow a bike for a gentle potter around the country lanes. Every day there are stretch and warm-up classes you can join in or – as you get a little fitter – toning and firming exercises. For the fairly fit, there's gymn equipment circuit training. Outdoors again, you can play badminton, tennis or croquet and horse-riding can be arranged. Try to keep 5 pm free – this is when the relaxation classes are held. Don't try to pack too much into your first couple of days – enjoy the luxury of unwinding and not having much to do. Don't worry if you feel sleepy for the first day or so. Enjoy an afternoon nap even if it means skipping one of the classes. If you're on a strict diet, you may have a headache for the first 24 hours so try to spend time outdoors just lounging around, without attempting anything too energetic.

## Won't the evenings seem long?
Most of us aren't used to leisurely evenings with no meals to cook, no long journey home, no quick drink

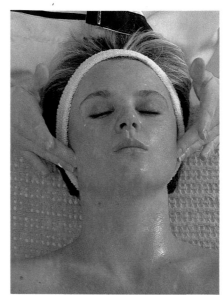
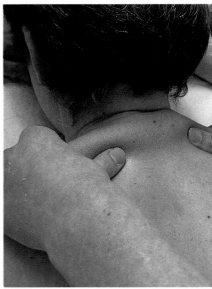
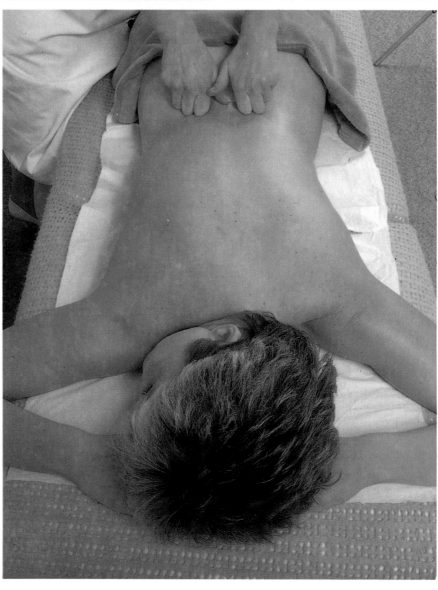

*Enjoy the wonderful pampered feeling that massage gives – so relaxing; it takes away all your stresses.*

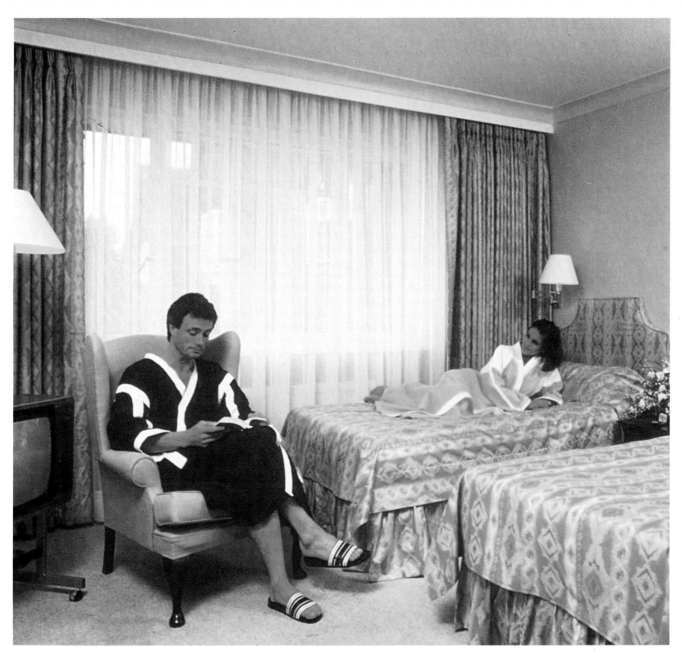

at the pub. But a good health farm makes sure that every hour is occupied (if you so wish) so after dinner you'll find something going on – a talk about antique furniture or art, live piano music in the drawing room, a bridge party or a Trivial Pursuit competition. No one stays up late because the combination of fresh air, exercise and good food makes you sleepy, but there's always a 'late night' video feature film shown around 9pm and, of course, if you really care what's happening in the outside world, each bedroom has television.

## Would it be OK to go alone?

While *Woman's Own* were visiting, there were married couples, businessmen taking a break alone, two secretaries who'd opted for a healthy week away from it all rather than a package holiday in Spain, three mums who'd arrived separately but soon became friends and a group of young footballers in need of some toning up. There's always someone to talk to. The staff are friendly, helpful and understanding – and the atmosphere is very relaxing.

If you possibly can, do try a

*Rooms are extremely comfortable with T.V. telephone and private bathroom.*

health farm break. The long-term effects will last you longer than a seaside holiday and, even when you're back into a more stressful lifestyle, you'll have learnt some new approaches to eating and exercise that will, hopefully, stay with you for the rest of your life.

*For details of health farms in Britain, Europe, Australia and the USA see pages 182 and 183.*

# Health farm directory

**Health farms in Britain**

**Brooklands Country House Health Farm,** Calder House Lane, Garstang, Preston, Lancashire (09952 5162). Luxury facilities, indoor pool, Turkish steam room, tennis courts. Prices include five daily treatments.

**Cedar Falls,** Bishops Lydeard, Taunton, Somerset (0823 433233). Set in a 40-acre/16ha estate surrounded by woods, trout fishing lakes, a par three golf course, there is a variety of beauty treatments and specialist programmes of aromatherapy, acupuncture and reflexology. Indoor pool, jacuzzi. Prices include four daily treatments.

**Champneys,** Tring, Hertfordshire (04427 73155). Medically supervised dieting and exercises. Relaxation classes, sports, luxury rooms, indoor pool, whirlpool and outdoor jacuzzi.

**Ellel Grange Health Hydro,** Ellel, Nr Lancaster, Lancashire (0524 752026). Luxury facilities, sauna, hydrotherapy bath, indoor pool, outdoor activities including horseriding. Four daily treatments included.

**Elm Farm Health Clinic,** Fulbrook, Burford, Oxfordshire (099382 3220). Small, exclusive clinic set in the beautiful Cotswolds. Luxury facilities. Prices include three daily treatments. Seven-day, three-day, weekend breaks or one-day visits.

**Enton Hall,** Enton, Nr Godalming, Surrey (042879 2233). Osteopathy and physiotherapy, specialized counselling for stress, variety of beauty treatments, outdoor pool.

**Forest Mere,** Liphook, Hampshire (0428 722051). Skin treatments and solarium, indoor and outdoor pools, physiotherapy.

**Grayshott Hall Health Centre,** Hindhead, Surrey (042873 4331). Luxury facilities, excellent diets and exercises. Indoor pool, nine-hole golf course and tennis courts. Prices include consultation and two treatments.

**Henlow Grange Health Farm,** Henlow, Bedfordshire (0462 811111). Beauty treatments, body massage, indoor pool, sauna.

**Imperial Health Club,** The Imperial Hotel, Torquay (0803 24301). Indoor pool, solarium, sauna, beauty and cosmetic treatments, low-calorie diets. Minimum three-day stay.

**Inglewood Health Hydro,** Kintbury, Newbury, Berkshire (0488 82022). Luxury stately home, medically supervised diets, beauty treatments, indoor pool.

**The Kingstone Clinic,** 291 Gilmerton Road, Edinburgh (031664 3435). Centre for naturopathic healing, offering vegetarian diets, exercise and massage.

**Maesteilo Mansion,** Capel Isaac, Llandeilo, Dyfed (05584 510). Specialized treatments include acupuncture, hypnosis, physiotherapy, plus a variety of beauty treatments and outdoor pool. All included in the price.

**The Primrose Hill Hydro,** St Saviour, Jersey (0534 26233). Luxury facilities, indoor pool, Californian whirlpool. Some treatments included in price.

**Ragdale Hall Health Hydro,** Ragdale, Nr Melton Mowbray, Leicestershire (0664 75831). Luxurious stately home, beautifully prepared slimming menus (and à la carte), wide range of beauty treatments, aromatherapy, indoor and outdoor pools, sports facilities. Open seven days a week.

**Shenley Lodge Health Resort,** Ridge Hill, Shenley, Radlett, Hertfordshire (0707 42424). Special weight-reducing or keep-fit courses. Programme based on high-protein diet combined with exercise, massage and sauna, daily courses are available too.

**Shrubland Hall Health Clinic,** Coddenham, Nr Ipswich, Suffolk (0473 830404). Gracious old country house, providing diets, beauty treatments, relaxation classes. Price includes two daily treatments.

**Tyringham Clinic,** Newport Pagnell, Buckinghamshire (0908 610450). Naturopathic treatments only. No beauty treatments. Prices include two treatments. Single rooms, twin-bedded and dormitory.

*Note* Some health farms offer one-day visits so you can sample treatments before you decide to book for a longer stay.

## Health farms in Europe

**Atsitsa,** Skyros Island, Greece. Contact: Penny Wise, 1 Fawley Road, London NW6 1SL (01-431 0867). Set on the beautiful Greek Island of Skyros, Atsitsa is known as 'the alternative health farm holiday' because it specializes in natural therapy and holistic healing. They have a variety of activities for you to try like windsurfing and other water sports as well as the more conventional exercise classes and for the mind and body there's T'ai Chi, yoga and meditation. Art and craft classes can be arranged for residents too.

**Brisamer S.L. Health and Beauty Farm,** Fuente de Perro, Apartado 34, Alhaurin el Grande, Malaga, Spain (01034 52 490891). Run by Leida Costigan, one of Europe's pioneers in health and beauty farms. There are a wide variety of beauty treatments and exercise classes available. Plus special diet consultations for those who want to lose weight. Brisamer has an outdoor pool and you can choose between staying in the luxury main house or their cheaper, but homely, garden chalets.

**Health Farm, Malta.** Contact: Halcyon Daze Ltd., Upper Farm, Kimbolton, Leominster, Herefordshire, UK (0568 87258). This is a value-for-money health farm holiday. Prices for a one week stay include flight, accommodation, full board, use of facilities, plus two treatments.

## Health farms in Australia

**Camp Eden,** Currumbin Creek Road, Currumbin Valley, Queensland (075 33 0111). Accommodation set in 250 acres/101 ha. This holistic health care retreat offers a wide range of beauty treatments and facilities including tennis courts, a swimming pool, massage, sauna, chiropractice, hydrotherapy, steam treatments, yoga and T'ai Chi. Personal advice given on losing weight and how to cope with stress.

**Dunn's Herbal Health Farm,** 10 Scarborough Beach Road, Scarborough, Western Australian (341 6788). With the accent on health, herbs and nutrition, Dunn's offers awareness weekends, cleansing, weekends, smoking and weight programme weekends, as well as relaxation therapy, individual food tests and diet plans.

**Hopewood Health Centre,** Greendale Road, Wallacia, New South Wales (047 73 8401). Lose weight safely and surely in peaceful surroundings under the guidance of qualified practioners. Relax and tone body and mind with natural foods, sunshine and a variety exercises.

**Solar Spring,** Contact: Suite 116, 160 Castlereagh Street, Sydney, New South Wales (264 9777). Health and fitness country club with resident naturopath, osteopath, dietician and beautician. Facilities include an indoor swimming pool, sauna, spa, solarium and massage. Bush walks, horse riding, archery, tennis and cyling provide additional exercise.

## Health farms in the USA

**The Aurora House Spa,** 35 East Garfield Road, Aurora, Ohio 44202, USA (0101 216 562 9171). Luxury 'Victorian' setting – has the latest in health/beauty equipment and facilities for both men and women. Very personal service for maximum of 30 guests.

**Carmel Country Spa,** 10 Country Club Way, Carmel Valley, California 93924 (0101 408 659 3798). This luxurious Californian country health farm is famous for its combined specialized weight loss and exercise programme where you can lose 1 lb/½ kg a day under strict medical supervision. Beauty treatments are extra and not included in the price because their main aim is successful weight loss.

**Golden Door,** P.O. Box 1567, Escondido, California 92025 (0101 619 744 5777). One of the most famous health spas in the USA, it offers a unique regime for health and beauty where your day begins with a mountain hike before breakfast and ends with a mini-massage in the Japanese bathhouse before bedtime. Guests are treated as equals – identities are put aside and housewives rub shoulders with heiresses unknowingly.

**The Spa at Palm-Aire,** 2501 Palm-Aire Drive, North Pompano Beach, Florida 33369 (0101 305 975 6122). Luxurious resort, maximum number of guests – 100. Variety of treatments and wide range of facilities including five golf courses, 37 tennis courts.

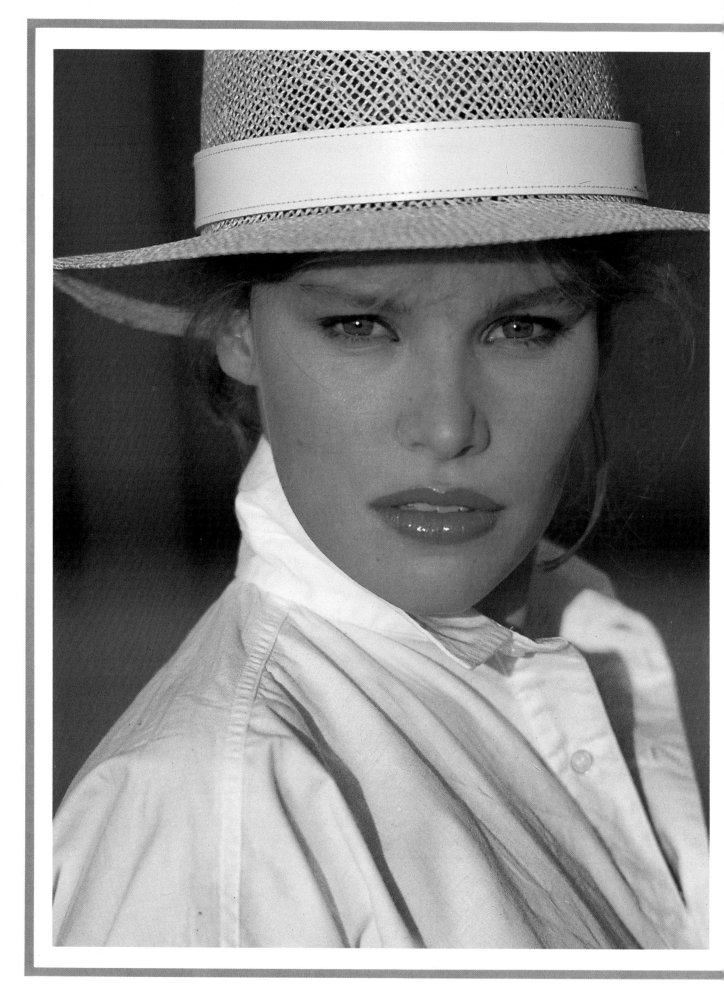

# Acknowledgements

Special thanks to photographer Rob Lee who shot the picture that appears opposite. His pictures also appear on pages 6, 11, 13, 15, 20, 23, 24, 29, 30, 31, 32, 33, 34, 35, 36, 37, 40, 41, 47, 50, 51, 52, 55, 59, 61, 84, 85, 90, 98, 101, 109, 113, 121, 122, 124, 126, 129, 131, 132, 139, 145, 153, 155, 161, 165, 166, 176, 177, 178 and 180.

*Other photographs by:*
John Adriaan, pages 56, 116, 159; Henry Arden, pages 77, 78, 79; David Barnes, pages 107, 108, 110, 127; Robert Belton, page 167; Nick Carmen, pages 68, 69, 86; John Carter, pages 42-3, 44, 45, 146; Roger Charity, page 46; Monty Coles, pages 27, 162; Alex James, page 46, 138; Nigel Limb, pages 72, 148, 173; Stefano Massimo, pages 123, 171; Malcolm Pasley, page 130; Helen Putsman, page 93; Otto Rauser, page 17, 91, 103; Christos Raftopoulos, page 81; David Steen, page 135; Peter Waldman, pages 16, 18, 24, 28, 99; Peter Underwood, page 114; Victor Yuan, page 89.
Photograph of Isabella Rossellini on page 119 by courtesy of Lancôme; photograph of Joan Collins on page 128 by courtesy of Revlon; photograph on page 137 by John Swannell courtesy of Ambre Solaire; photographs on pages 141, 143, 149 by Ken Browar by courtesy of L'Oreal Keratase Nutritive; photograph of Sophia Loren on page 133 and accompanying text copyright © Scelo Enterprises, N.V. 1984.
Photograph on page 168 Hamlyn Publishing Group Limited; photographs on pages 175, 181 by courtesy of Grayshott Hall.

*Illustrations*
Kevin Madison, pages 40, 70, 71, 83, 87;
Lucy Su, pages 21, 25, 39.
Facial massage technique on page 25 by courtesy of Elizabeth Arden.

Thanks to *Women's Own* staff – Norma Knox, Angela Covington, Petsa Kaffens, Lyn Walford, Mitzi Wilson (for supplying additional pictures and copy) and to Dorothy Sims for keeping everything in its proper place! Thanks also to Annie Anderson and hairdresser Annie Russell.

Designer: JO TAPPER
Copy editor: SALLY WOOD ·

# Index

*Page numbers in italics indicate illustrations*